Handbook of Thromboprophylaxis

Second edition

Handbook of Thromboprophylaxis
Second edition

David Perry (Editor)
Addenbrooke's Hospital, Cambridge, UK

David Warwick
Southampton University Hospitals, Southampton, UK

David Gozzard
Betsi Cadwaladr University Health Board, North Wales, UK

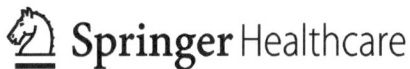 Springer Healthcare

Published by Springer Healthcare, 236 Gray's Inn Road, London, WC1X 8HB, UK

www.currentmedicinegroup.com

British Library Cataloguing-in-Publication Data.

A catalogue record for this book is available from the British Library.

ISBN 978-1-907673-09-2

Although every effort has been made to ensure that drug doses and other information are presented accurately in this publication, the ultimate responsibility rests with the prescribing physician. Neither the publisher nor the authors can be held responsible for errors or for any consequences arising from the use of the information contained herein. Any product mentioned in this publication should be used in accordance with the prescribing information prepared by the manufacturers. No claims or endorsements are made for any drug or compound at present under clinical investigation.

Project editor: Anne Carty
Designer: Joe Harvey
Typesetting: Sissan Mollerfors
Production: Marina Maher

Contents

Author biographies

David Perry MD, PLD, FRCPEdin, FRCPath, is Consultant in Haemostasis, Thrombosis and General Haematology at Addenbrooke's Hospital, Cambridge, UK, an Honorary Lecturer at the University of Cambridge, and Co-Director of the Haemophilia Comprehensive Care Centre. Prior to joining the staff at Addenbrooke's Hospital, he was Senior Lecturer in Haemostasis and Thrombosis at the Royal Free and University College Medical School (Royal Free Campus), London, UK. His interests include the molecular genetics of haemostasis and thrombosis, the rare inherited bleeding disorders and the management of patients with venous thromboembolic disease, particularly in relation to pregnancy. He has published widely in the area of haemostasis and thrombosis. He is a member of the British Committee for Standards in Haematology Task Force on Haemostasis & Thrombosis, a member of the steering group for UK National External Quality Assessment Service (Blood Coagulation) and chairs the Specialist Advisory Group for Haemophilia Molecular Genetics for UK National External Quality Assessment Service. His other interests include medical education – he is examiner for the Royal College of Physicians, Edinburgh and the Royal College of Pathologists and is the current lead physician for pathology education at Addenbrooke's Hospital.

David Warwick MD, FRCS, FRCS(Orth), is Reader in Orthopaedic Surgery at Southampton University Hospitals, UK. He has been researching orthopaedic thromboembolism since 1991. This work led to a Hunterian Professorship at the Royal College of Surgeons and a doctorate from the University of Bristol. He has published 19 papers on thromboembolism in peer-reviewed journals, has written several invited articles and has presented at many national and international meetings. He is a co-author of the THRIFT guidelines (1998), and the International Consensus Statement (2001, 2006). He was Chairman of the International Surgical Thrombosis Forum Guidelines Group. He reviews papers on orthopaedic thrombosis for the *Journal of Bone and Joint Surgery* and is co-author of the latest edition of *Apley's System of Orthopaedics*. He lectures regularly on orthopaedic thromboembolism in Britain and abroad. He has been an Invited Instructor at the American Academy of Orthopaedic Surgeons and a Witness to the UK Parliamentary Enquiry into Thromboembolism. He presently sits on the National Institute for Clinical Excellence Orthopaedic VTE Guidelines Development Group.

David Gozzard FRCP, FRCPath, MBA is Consultant Haematologist and former Medical Director at the North Wales NHS trust in North Wales. He has a career-long interest in coagulation and has been actively involved in thromboprophylaxis strategies around indwelling long-line catheters in the on-site North Wales Cancer Treatment Centre. He was the clinical executive lead for the Safer Patient Initiative, a UK collaboration with the Institute for Healthcare Improvement, Boston, USA, and the Health Foundation. Under his clinical leadership the trust has gained a significant reputation in the field of patient safety. As Medical Director, he is actively involved in modernisation as the executive lead and has developed considerable experience in clinical leadership, change management and policy implementation in the clinical professions. In 2007 he was successful in obtaining a fellowship award from the Health Foundation to allow him to study with the Institute for Healthcare Improvement in Boston for 12 months.

Abbreviations

ACCP	American College of Chest Physicians
APS	antiphospholipid syndrome
ARTEMIS	Arixtra for ThromboEmbolism prevention in Medical Indications Study
BMI	body mass index
CI	confidence interval
DVT	deep vein thrombosis
ENDORSE	Epidemiologic International Day for the Evaluation of Outcomes Research
ENOXACAN	ENOXAparin in CANcer
FRONTLINE	Fundamental Research in Oncology and Thrombosis
GCS	graduated compression stockings
GECS	graduated elastic compression stockings
INR	international normalised ratio
IPC	intermittent pneumatic compression
LMWH	low-molecular-weight heparin
MEDENOX	incidence of VTE in the MEDical patients with ENOXaparin
MI	myocardial infarction
NR	not recommended
NYHA	New York Health Association
PE	pulmonary embolism
PNH	paroxysmal nocturnal haemogloburinia
PREVENT	Prospective Evaluation of Dalteparin Efficacy for Prevention of VTE in Immobilised Patients
PRIME	Prophylaxis in Internal Medicine with Enoxaparin
THE-PRINCE	Thromboembolism Prevention in Cardiac or Respiratory Disease with Enoxaparin
QALY	quality-adjusted life-years
RCT	randomised controlled trial
RR	risk reduction
SCI	spinal cord injury
SIGN	Scottish Intercollegiate Guidelines Network
TEDS	thromboembolism deterrent stockings
THR	total hip replacement
THRIFT	Thromboembolic Risk Factors Trial

TKR	total knee replacement
UFH	unfractionated heparin
VFP	venous foot pump
VKA	vitamin K antagonist
VTE	venous thromboembolism

Chapter 1

Introduction

This *Handbook of Thromboprophylaxis* expands upon the role of anticoagulants in clinical practice. We have attempted to summarise key papers in the field and to provide evidence-based guidelines for their use in routine day-to-day practice.

There is an increasing awareness of the risks of venous thromboembolic disease, which includes deep vein thrombosis (DVT) and pulmonary embolism (PE). In the UK, this was quite clearly highlighted by the publication of the *Health Committee's report on the Prevention of Venous Thromboembolism in Hospitalised Patients* in 2005 [1], the *Department of Health (DoH) Independent Working Group report on the Prevention of Venous Thromboembolism in Hospitalised Patients* [2] in 2007 the *National Institute of Health and Clinical Excellence (NICE) guidelines on surgical patients* [3] published in 2010.

Each year, over 25,000 people in England die from venous thromboembolism (VTE) that develops in hospital – a figure that is more than the combined total of deaths from breast cancer, AIDS and traffic accidents, and more than 25 times the number who die from methicillin-resistant *Staphylococcus aureus* (MRSA).

Despite the high risk of VTE in hospitalised patients and the undoubted benefit of pharmacological thromboprophylaxis, many patients do not receive any form of thromboprophylaxis. A fundamental change to our approach to the management of all hospitalised patients is required. All of our patients should undergo assessment of their risk of VTE on admission. Rather than ask 'does this patient merit thromboprophylaxis?', we should establish 'are there reasons for not prescribing pharmacological thromboprophylaxis in this patient?' This is a key recommendation of both the DoH Working Group report and the NICE guidelines.

The DoH recommends that all patients undergo risk assessment for VTE on admission to hospital. In addition, patients should be reassessed periodically after at least 48–72 hours during their inpatient stage, as their level of risk may change [4]. Figure 1.1 shows the DoH assessment sheet for VTE.

DoH assessment sheet for DVT		
	Patient related	**Procedure related**
Thrombosis risk		
High	Age >60 years	Hip or knee replacement
	Previous pulmonary embolism or deep vein thrombosis	Hip fracture
	Active cancer	Other major othropaedic surgery
	Acute or chronic inflammatory disease	
	Chronic heart failure	
	Lower limb paralysis (excluding acute stroke)	
	Acute infectious disease, eg pneumonia	
	BMI >30 kg/m^2	
Moderate		Surgical procedure lasting >30 minutes
		Plaster cast immobilisation of lower limb
Bleeding risk		
	Haemophilia or other known bleeding disorder	Neurosurgery, spinal surgery or eye surgery
	Known platelet count <100	Other procedure with high bleeding risk
	Acute stroke in previous month (haemorrhagic or ischaemic)	Lumbar puncture/spinal/epidural in previous 4 hours
	Blood pressure >200 systolic or 120 diastolic	
	Severe liver disease (prothrombin time above normal or known varices)	
	Severe renal disease	
	Active bleeding	
	Major bleeding risk, existing anticoagulant therapy or antiplatelet therapy	

Figure 1.1 Adapted from DoH assessment sheet for DVT [4].

Finally, VTE is costly and it is estimated that the annual cost in the UK for treating patients with post-surgical VTE is in the region of £204 million to £228 million, and the total cost to the UK for the management of VTE is estimated at £640 million. Simple measures can improve the health of patients and has the potential to significantly reduce the cost of healthcare in the UK.

References

1. House of Commons Health Committee. The prevention of venous thromboembolism in hospitalised patients. Second report of session 2004–5. Available at: www.publications.parliament.uk/pa/cm200405/cmselect/cmhealth/99/99.pdf.
2. Department of Health. Report of the independent expert working group on the prevention of venous thromboembolism in hospitalised patients. Smart No. 278330 (April 2007). Available at: www.dh.gov.uk/en/Publicationsandstatistics/Publications/PublicationsPolicyAndGuidance/DH_073944.
3. National Institute of Clinical Excellence. Venous thromboembolism–reducing the risk. NICE clinical guidelines CG92 (January 2010). Available at: www.nice.org.uk/nicemedia/pdf/CG92NICEGuidance.pdf.
4. Department of Health. Risk assessment for venous thromboembolism (VTE). Gateway reference No. 10278 (September 2008). Available at: www.dh.gov.uk/en/Publicationsandstatistics/Publications/PublicationsPolicyAndGuidance/DH_088215.

Chapter 2

Thromboprophylaxis in medical patients

Introduction

Venous thromboembolic (VTE) disease is a significant cause of morbidity and mortality in hospitalised patients. The acutely ill or nonsurgical 'medical' patient represents approximately 60% of all hospital admissions in the UK and such patients are at high risk of VTE. Postmortem data suggest that approximately 10% of deaths that occur in hospitals are due to pulmonary embolism (PE) [1–3].

In the absence of thromboprophylaxis, the incidence of VTE in the MEDical patients with ENOXaparin (MEDENOX) study [4] was 14.9% and for proximal deep vein thrombosis (DVT) alone 4.9%. The incidence of VTE in the control arm of the Prospective Evaluation of Dalteparin Efficacy for Prevention of VTE in Immobilised Patients (PREVENT) trial was 4.96% [5] and in the Arixtra® (fondaparinux) for ThromboEmbolism prevention in Medical Indications Study (ARTEMIS) 10.5% for all VTE [6].

Data from the large-scale Epidemiologic International Day for the Evaluation of Outcomes Research (ENDORSE) study have more recently shown that 42% of medical inpatients are at risk of VTE but that less than half (40%) receive appropriate preventative treatment [7].

VTE is largely preventable and prophylaxis with low-molecular-weight heparins (LMWHs) has been shown to be well-tolerated and cost-effective in numerous studies involving surgical patients. Over the past decade a large number of well-conducted, prospective, randomised trials have consistently demonstrated that the appropriate use of pharmacological thromboprophylaxis can significantly reduce the risk of VTE in medical patients. There is accumulating evidence that use of thromboprophylaxis with LMWHs in this group of patients is both safe and effective. Three key trials involving medical patients – MEDENOX, PREVENT and ARTEMIS – have shown a relative risk reduction of DVT of 50–65% with the appropriate use of thromboprophylaxis (LMWHs or fondaparinux).

A key issue that remains to be resolved, however, is the duration of thromboprophylaxis in medical patients [8]. Data from trials involving surgical patients suggest that the risk of thrombosis persists for several weeks and such patients may require extended out-of-hospital thromboprophylaxis.

Risk factors and risk assessment models in medical patients

Hospitalised medical patients are often at increased risk of VTE because of the presence of one or more factors. These factors are outlined in Figure 2.1.

Medical patients may also vary in their susceptibility to VTE. For example, a large pulmonary embolus may be asymptomatic in an otherwise healthy mobile individual but may prove fatal if a patient has a low cardiopulmonary reserve.

In light of these evidence- and consensus-based risk factors, a number of risk models have been proposed. A risk assessment model for medical thromboprophylaxis should ideally:

- identify medical patients who are at significant risk of VTE and who would, therefore, benefit from thromboprophylaxis;
- identify patients with contraindications to thromboprophylaxis or who would not benefit from thromboprophylaxis;
- allow transparent and simple decision making at the bedside; and
- be evidence based.

A simplified risk assessment model was proposed by Cohen et al. [9] that can be applied to all medical patients (Figure 2.2). It revolves around the following two decisions:

1. 'Is the patient at increased risk of VTE?' If the answer is yes, they should be considered for thromboprophylaxis.

Risk factors for VTE in hospitalised medical patients	
History of DVT or PE	Stroke
Family history of VTE	Prolonged immobility (>4 days)
Acute infection	Acute or chronic lung disease
Malignancy	Acute inflammatory disease
Age (>75 years)	Inflammatory bowel disease
Congestive heart failure	Shock
Paraproteinaemia	Hyperhomocysteinaemia
Behçet's disease	Dysfibrinogenaemia
Nephrotic syndrome	Myeloproliferative disorders
Hypofibrinolysis	Age (>41 years)
Polycythaemia	Sepsis (<1 month)
PNH	Heparin-induced thrombocytopenia
High-dose oestrogen therapy	Congenital or acquired thrombophilia
Obesity (BMI ≥30 kg/m²)	Varicose veins

Figure 2.1 BMI, body mass index; DVT, deep vein thrombosis; PE, pulmonary embolism; PNH, paroxysmal nocturnal haemogloburinia; VTE, venous thromboembolism.

2. 'Is pharmacological thromboprophylaxis contraindicated?' If the answer is yes, other forms of thromboprophylaxis, such as mechanical thrombo-prophylaxis, should be considered. If the answer is no, pharmacological thromboprophylaxis is indicated.

This risk assessment model is applicable to all patients over the age of 40 years who have both evidence- or consensus-based acute medical illnesses and reduced mobility. It also takes into account patients' specific predisposing risk factors. Implementation of this simple risk assessment model would considerably increase the uptake of thromboprophylaxis in acutely medically ill patients and significantly reduce the burden of VTE.

Thromboprophylaxis clinical trials in medical patients

There have been three large prospective randomised placebo-controlled studies of LMWHs versus placebo performed in recent years. In 1999, the MEDENOX study [4] was published comparing enoxaparin in two doses (20 mg or 40 mg) against placebo. Subsequently, the PREVENT study [5], comparing dalteparin with placebo, and the ARTEMIS study [6], comparing the synthetic pentasaccharide fondaparinux with placebo, were published in 2004 and 2006 respectively. In addition, an analysis of combined data from the OASIS 5 and 6 trials comparing fondaparinux with a heparin-based strategy was published in 2008. A number of smaller trials have also compared LMWHs, primarily enoxaparin, with unfractionated heparins (UFHs) and have been analysed in a meta-analysis [10].

The MEDENOX study followed 866 acutely ill medical patients for 14 days with bilateral ascending venography to determine the incidence of VTE and the efficacy of enoxaparin as treatment [4]. Two doses of enoxaparin were evaluated, 20 mg subcutaneously once daily and 40 mg subcutaneously once daily. The low dose produced results that were not significantly different from placebo, whereas the higher dose resulted in a 63% relative risk reduction in all VTE ($p<0.001$) and a 65% relative risk reduction ($p=0.04$) in proximal DVT. This significant reduction in the incidence of VTE was shown to be safe with no significant increase in major haemorrhagic adverse effects. Subgroup analysis of the MEDENOX study showed efficacy in all major clinical groups [11].

The ARTEMIS study assessed the incidence and treatment of VTE in 849 (425 patients in the fondaparinux group and 414 patients in the placebo group – 10 were not evaluated) acutely ill medical patients. The primary efficacy outcome was the incidence of VTE up to day 15 and treatment with fondaparinux was given in a dose of 2.5 mg subcutaneously once daily, similar to that used in high-risk surgical procedures. This study showed an incidence

Risk assessment model for VTE in medical patients

All medical patients should be routinely assessed and considered for thromboprophylaxis

Is the patient >40 years old with acute medical illness and reduced mobility?

Yes | **No**

Does the patient have one of the following acute medical illnesses/conditions? Evidence based*:
• Acute MI
• Acute heart failure NYHA III/IV
• Acute cancer requiring therapy
• Acute infectious disease (including severe infection/sepsis)
• Respiratory disease (respiratory failure with/without mechanical ventilation, exacerbations of chronic respiratory disease)
• Rheumatic disease (including acute arthritis of lower extremities and vertebral compression)
• Ischaemic stroke†
• Paraplegia

Consensus view only:
• Inflammatory disorder with immobility
• Inflammatory bowel disease

Yes | **No**

Is pharmacological thromboprophylaxis contraindicated?

Yes Does the patient‡ have one of the following risk factors? Evidence based in acutely ill medical patients §
• History of VTE
• History of malignancy
• Age >75 years

Consensus based from strong evidence in other settings:
• Prolonged immobility
• Age >60 years
• Varicose veins
• Obesity
• Hormone therapy
• Pregnancy/postpartum
• Nephrotic syndrome
• Dehydration
• Thrombophillia
• Thrombocytosis

Yes | **No** | **No**

| Mechanical thromboprophylaxis with graduated compression stockings or intermittent pneumatic compression is recommended ¥ | LMWH (enoxaparin 40 mg o.d. or dalteparin 5000 IU o.d.) or UFH (5000 IU q8h) (LMWH preferred due to better safety profile) | No evidence for the benefits of thromboprophylaxis. However, patients should be considered for thromboprophylaxis on a case-by-case basis |

Figure 2.2 *Equivalent to the evidence used by the American College of Chest Physicians for a Grade 1A recommendation (outlined in Chapter 4). †Note: the patient's risk of haemorrhagic transformation should be assessed before giving thromboprophylaxis. ‡Medical outpatients whose acute medical illness is not included in the risk assessment model should be considered for thromboprophylaxis on a case-by-case basis depending on the severity of their acute medical illness and their risk factors. §Evidence based primarily on subanalyses of the MEDENOX study. ¥Based on generalizations from randomised trials in other patient groups. LMWH, low-molecular-weight heparin; MI, myocardial infarction; NYHA, New York Health Association; o.d., once daily; UFH, unfractionated heparin; VTE, venous thromboembolism. Reproduced with permission from Cohen et al. [9].

of VTE in the placebo group of 10.5%, with a 46.7% odds reduction with treatment (p=0.029) [6].

The PREVENT study compared dalteparin 5000 IU subcutaneously once daily against placebo in 3706 acute medically ill patients. The cohort of acutely ill medical patients consisted of 52% with chronic heart failure and 30% with respiratory failure; the remaining patients had infection without septic shock, rheumatic disorders or inflammatory bowel disease. The study used ultrasound (in contrast to the MEDENOX and ARTEMIS studies, which employed venography) to detect proximal venous thrombosis and was, therefore, unable to detect distal calf thrombosis unless the patient was symptomatic, probably resulting in an underestimation of the true incidence of distal DVT. However, the incidence of proximal venous thrombosis in the placebo group was lower at 5%. The incidence of VTE in the treated group was 2.8% (p=0.0015), with a similar risk reduction in both asymptomatic proximal DVT and symptomatic DVT [12].

Mehta et al. conducted an individual patient-level combined analysis of 26,512 patients with ST- and non-ST-segment elevation acute coronary syndromes from the OASIS 5 and 6 trials, who were randomised to fonda-parinux 2.5 mg daily or a heparin-based strategy (dose-adjusted unfraction-ated heparin or enoxaparin). This showed that fondaparinux was superior to heparin in reducing the composite of death, myocardial infarction or stroke, at 7.2% versus 8.0% and a hazard ratio of 0.91. The risk of death alone was also significantly reduced with fondaparinux versus heparin, at 3.8% versus 4.3% and a hazard ratio of 0.89, as was the risk of major bleeding, at 3.4% versus 2.1% and a hazard ratio of 0.9. Overall, patients receiving fondaparinux had a significantly more favourable clinical outcome than patients in the heparin arm, at a hazard ratio of 0.83 [13].

The magnitude of the risk reduction is broadly consistent across all three of these studies and equates approximately to the 50–65% relative risk reduction seen in the incidence of VTE following high-risk orthopaedic surgery, such as elective primary hip and knee replacement surgery. A meta-analysis comparing heparin – both UFH and LMWH – with placebo as thromboprophylaxis in medical patients [10] found a significant reduction in DVT and pulmonary embolus when using heparin, and a non-significant increase in haemor-rhage. Another meta-analysis also compared LMWH with UFH and showed a trend of improved efficacy of LMWH over UFH in the treatment of DVT. More importantly, it showed a significant reduction in major haemorrhage in LMWH compared with UFH; therefore, while both treatments are efficacious, LMWH is the safer. However, all three of the above prospective randomised trials demonstrated the safety of pharmacological thromboprophylaxis in general in acutely ill medical patients.

The safety of LMWH was evident in the Thromboembolism Prevention in Cardiac or Respiratory Disease with Enoxaparin (THE-PRINCE) study [14], which was a multicentre, randomised, open, parallel-group study that compared subcutaneous enoxaparin 40 mg subcutaneously once daily with UFH 5000 IU three times daily for the prevention of VTE in patients with heart failure or severe respiratory disease. There was no difference in efficacy between the two treatment groups, although bleeding events were less frequent in patients receiving enoxaparin (1.5%) than in the UFH arm (3.6%). Similar results were found in the Prophylaxis in Internal Medicine with Enoxaparin (PRIME) study [15], which compared the safety and efficacy of enoxaparin with UFH in 959 patients hospitalised as a result of acute medical illness and with at least one additional risk factor for VTE.

A meta-analysis of the safety of thromboprophylaxis in acute medical illness [16] evaluated data from 2346 patients. Similar rates of major bleeding (about 1%) were observed in patients given enoxaparin, UFH or placebo. The incidence of minor bleeding was comparable in the enoxaparin and placebo groups but significantly higher in the group receiving UFH compared with enoxaparin. These data are in contrast to the meta-analysis conducted by Mismetti et al. [10], which reported a significantly lower rate of major bleeding in medical patients receiving LMWH.

The combined results of these various trials highlight that medical patients are at high risk of VTE when immobilised with acute medical illnesses, and this risk can be reduced by the use of pharmacological prophylaxis with LMWH. The magnitude of the risk reduction with LMWH is similar to that seen in high-risk orthopaedic surgery using a comparable dose of UFH. Lower doses of LMWH do not appear to be more efficacious than placebo. As a result of the evidence provided by analysis of these studies, a number of national and international guidelines for the use of pharmacological thromboprophylaxis in medical patients have become available. Medical thromboprophylaxis is a Grade 1 recommendation in the American College of Chest Physicians (ACCP) guidelines [17] and is recommended in both the Scottish and Intercollegiate Guideline Network (SIGN) [18] and the Thromboembolic Risk Factors (THRIFT II) consensus group guidelines [19]. NICE recommend that pharmacological thromboprophylaxis is offered to general medical patients who have been assessed as being at an increased risk of VTE. The can be in the form of fondaparinux, LMWH or UFH. This should start as soon as possible after risk assessment and should continue until the patient is no longer at increased risk of VTE. [20] These guidelines all recommend the use of pharmacological thromboprophylaxis in acutely ill medical patients in whom there is no contraindication.

More recent recommendations were set out in the report by the Department of Health (DoH) Working Group on Venous Thromboembolism [21], which states that all medical patients should undergo mandatory risk assessment and should be considered for thromboprophylaxis. LMWH is the preferred prophylactic approach. Mechanical means of thromboprophylaxis are not currently recommended due to lack of sufficient data in acutely ill patients, and aspirin is not recommended at all as a form of thromboprophylaxis in medical patients.

Who should not receive thromboprophylaxis?

While there is now substantial evidence that pharmacological thromboprophylaxis with LMWH in medical patients who are at high risk of VTE significantly reduces this risk and is not associated with significant adverse effects, a number of barriers to the implementation of medical thromboprophylaxis have been identified, including the need for a simple, widely applicable, risk assessment model. Other issues include concerns over the applicability of the available data [4–6] to all medical patients. However, the introduction of the risk assessment model described earlier should enable all medical patients to be evaluated for risk.

Several medical conditions exist that can complicate the treatment of a patient, including:

- recent surgery;
- a known bleeding disorder;
- impaired renal function with a creatinine clearance of <30 ml/min;
- uncontrolled hypertension;
- a recent ischaemic cerebral infarction; and
- active or a history of gastrointestinal bleeding.

In addition, the use of antiplatelet agents or non steroidal anti-inflammatory drugs may also raise concerns about bleeding with the concomitant use of a LMWH. Conversely, advancing age, active cancer, previous DVT, obesity with a body mass index (BMI) of more than 30 kg/m^2, active inflammatory infections, stroke with hemiplegia, chronic heart or respiratory failure, or hormone therapy, may place these patients at a greater risk of developing VTE than patients recruited into the clinical trials.

If contraindications to the use of pharmacological thromboprophylaxis in the acutely ill medical patient do exist, mechanical thromboprophylaxis with graduated compression stockings (GCS) or intermittent pneumatic compression (IPC) should be considered [17].

References

1. Cohen AT, Edmondson RA, Phillips MJ, et al. The changing pattern of venous thromboembolic disease. Haemostasis 1996; 26:65–71.
2. Lindblad B, Sternby NH, Bergqvist D. Incidence of venous thromboembolism verified by necropsy over 30 years. BMJ 1991; 302:709–711.
3. Sandler DA, Martin JF. Autopsy proven PE in hospital patients: are we detecting enough deep vein thrombosis? J R Soc Med 1989; 82:203–205.
4. Samama MM, Cohen AT, Darmon JY, et al. A comparison of enoxaparin with placebo for the prevention of venous thromboembolism in acutely ill medical patients. Prophylaxis in MEDical Patients with ENOXaparin Study Group. N Engl J Med 1999; 341:793–800.
5. Leizorovicz A, Cohen AT, Turpie AG, et al. Randomized, placebo-controlled trial of dalteparin for the prevention of venous thromboembolism in acutely ill medical patients. Circulation 2004; 110:874–879.
6. Cohen AT, Davidson BL, Gallus AS, et al. Efficacy and safety of fondaparinux for the prevention of venous thromboembolism in older acute medical patients: randomised placebo controlled trial. BMJ 2006; 332:325–329.
7. Cohen AT, Tapson VF, Bergmann JF, et al. A large-scale, global observational study of venous thromboembolism risk and prophylaxis in the acute hospital care setting: the ENDORSE study. J Thromb Haemostasis 2007; 1(Suppl 1):Abstract OS002.
8. Turpie AG. Extended duration of thromboprophylaxis in acutely ill medical patients: optimizing therapy? J Thromb Haemost 2007; 5:5–11.
9. Cohen AT, Alikhan R, Arcelus JI, et al. Assessment of venous thromboembolism risk and the benefits of thromboprophylaxis in medical patients. Thromb Haemost 2005; 94:750–759.
10. Mismetti P, Laporte-Simitsidis S, Tardy B, et al. Prevention of venous thromboembolism in internal medicine with unfractionated or low-molecular-weight heparins: a meta-analysis of randomised clinical trials. Thromb Haemost 2000; 83:14–19.
11. Alikhan R, Cohen AT, Combe S, et al. Prevention of venous thromboembolism in medical patients with enoxaparin: a subgroup analysis of the MEDENOX study. Blood Coagul Fibrinolysis 2003; 14:341–346.
12. Leizorovicz A, Cohen AT, Turpie AG, et al. Randomized, placebo-controlled trial of dalteparin for the prevention of venous thromboembolism in acutely ill medical patients. Circulation 2004; 110:874–879.
13. Mehta SR, Boden WE, Eikelboom JW, et al. Antithrombotic therapy with fondaparinux in relation to interventional management strategy in patients with ST- and non-ST-segment elevation acute coronary syndromes: an individual patient-level combined analysis of the Fifth and Sixth Organization to Assess Strategies in Ischemic Syndromes (OASIS 5 and 6) randomized trials. Circulation 2009; 118:2038–2046.
14. Kleber FX, Witt C, Vogel G, et al. THE-PRINCE Study Group. Randomized comparison of enoxaparin with unfractionated heparin for the prevention of venous thromboembolism in medical patients with heart failure or severe respiratory disease. Am Heart J 2003; 145:614–621.
15. Bergmann JF, Neuhart E. A multicenter randomized double-blind study of enoxaparin compared with unfractionated heparin in the prevention of venous thromboembolic disease in elderly in-patients bedridden for an acute medical illness. The Enoxaparin in Medicine Study Group. Thromb Haemost 1996; 76:529–534.
16. Alikhan R, Cohen AT. A safety analysis of thromboprophylaxis in acute medical illness. Thromb Haemost 2003; 89:590–591.
17. Geerts WH, Berqvist D, Pineo GF, et al. Prevention of venous thromboembolism. American College of Chest Physicians Evidence-Based Clinical Practice Guidelines. Chest 2008; 133(Suppl):381S–453S.
18. Scottish and Collegiate Guideline Network (SIGN). Prophylaxis of Venous Thromboembolism. London, SIGN publication, 2002; no. 62. Available at: www.sign.ac.uk/guidelines.

19. Thromboembolic Risk Factors (THRIFT II) Consensus Group Guidelines. Available at: www.clinicalconsensusreports.com.
20. National Institute of Clinical Excellence. Venous thromboembolism - reducing the risk NICE clinical guidelines CG92 (January 2010). Available at: www.nice.org.uk/nicemedia/pdf/CG92NICEGuidance.pdf.
21. Department of Health. Report of the independent expert working group on the prevention of venous thromboembolism in hospitalised patients. Smart No. 278330 (April 2007). Available at: www.dh.gov.uk/en/Publicationsandstatistics/Publications/PublicationsPolicyAndGuidance/DH_073944.

Chapter 3

Pharmacoeconomics of medical thromboprophylaxis

It is clear that medical patients are at increased risk of developing VTE, and such patients place significant demands upon healthcare systems due to high rates of hospitalisations and need for treatment. VTE is costly, although there is currently a paucity of data on the economics of medical thromboprophylaxis. It is estimated that the annual cost in the UK for treating patients with post surgical VTE lies in the region of £204 million to £228 million, and the total costs to the UK for the management of VTE is estimated at £640 million [1]. Simple measures can improve the health of our patients and have the potential to significantly reduce the cost of healthcare in the UK.

Bergqvist et al. [2] performed a retrospective cost analysis of clinical trial data, examining the healthcare costs incurred by 257 patients with a prior DVT of the lower limb versus 241 age- and gender-matched controls. Over an average follow-up of 10–15 years, there were 242 complications among patients with a previous DVT, compared with just 25 events in the control group, giving a tenfold increased risk of complications in the thrombosis arm. The majority of complications occurred within 5 years of the baseline DVT event. Furthermore, survival was markedly different at 35% in patients with a previous DVT versus 57% among controls. The total cost of treating patients with a previous DVT over 15 years was determined as SEK 7,850,696 (US$1,427,399) versus SEK 607,104 (US$110,383) for controls. This gave an average cost per complication of SEK 32,441 (US$5898) for thrombosis patients, compared with SEK 24,284 (US$4415) for controls.

In an economic evaluation of data from the MEDENOX trial [3] performed over an average follow-up of 90 days, the incidence of thromboembolic events was 5.5% with enoxaparin 40 mg versus 14.9% for placebo, and represented a substantial reduction in VTE. However, there were 16 deaths in the placebo arm and none in the enoxaparin 40 mg arm. The economic evaluation showed that the median cost per death avoided with enoxaparin 40 mg was €8102 (US$10,245), with a median cost per life-year gained of €2701 (US$3415) and a maximum cost of €17,757 (US$22,455), assuming a life expectancy of 3 years.

Three pharmacoeconomic studies have modelled the costs of VTE thromboprophylaxis in acutely ill medical patients [4–6]. Lloyd et al. [4] used a previously validated decision tree model based upon epidemiological data, clinical trials and a meta-analysis to evaluate the cost-effectiveness of enoxaparin (40 mg once daily) compared with either UFH (5000 IU twice daily) or no VTE thromboprophylaxis. Results were calculated for a hypothetical cohort of 100 patients. The expected cost per 100 patients was £9992, £9972 and £8781 with enoxaparin, UFH and no prophylaxis, respectively, and the expected number of episodes of VTE per 100 patients was 1.2, 1.4 and 3.2, respectively. The expected number of episodes of major bleeding per 100 patients was 1.7 with enoxaparin, 3.5 with UFH and 1.1 with no prophylaxis, and the cost-effectiveness ratio for enoxaparin compared to no prophylaxis was calculated as £796 per VTE event avoided. In summary, enoxaparin was found to be cost-effective compared with no thromboprophylaxis, although no benefit was seen between enoxaparin and thromboprophylaxis with UFH.

de Lissovoy et al. [5] looked at the cost effectiveness of adding VTE prophylaxis with enoxaparin to the standard care for acutely ill, hospitalised medical patients. They used a pharmacoeconomic model designed to simulate the 6- to 14-day course of enoxaparin prophylaxis evaluated in the MEDENOX trial. VTE prophylaxis with enoxaparin was estimated to account for 1.2–2.4% of the cost of a hospital admission, with an additional US$23±US$28 to US$99±US$122 to complete a course of out-of-hospital prophylaxis. Incremental cost effectiveness of VTE prophylaxis relative to no prophylaxis ranged from US$1249 to US$3088 per VTE avoided. The authors concluded that the use of thromboprophylaxis with enoxaparin in the acutely ill medical patient results in only a small increase in treatment costs; that prophylaxis is cost effective in terms of incremental cost per VTE avoided; and there is a reasonable probability that the cost of prophylaxis will be offset by avoided future VTE treatment.

McGarry et al. [6] used a decision tree model to estimate the cost effectiveness of VTE prophylaxis in a hypothetical cohort of 10,000 patients. Thromboprophylaxis comprised either enoxaparin 40 mg once daily or UFH 5000 IU twice daily, or no prophylaxis. The expected numbers of deaths attributable to VTE or drug complications related to prophylaxis for and treatment of VTE over a 30-day period were 37 with enoxaparin prophylaxis,

53 with UFH prophylaxis, and 81 with no prophylaxis. In 2001, the expected costs for prevention, diagnosis, and management of VTE were US$3,502,000, US$3,772,000 and US$3,105,000 for enoxaparin, UFH and no prophylaxis, respectively. The incremental cost per death averted with enoxaparin prophylaxis versus no prophylaxis was US$9100, and when compared with UFH, enoxaparin was less costly and more effective.

An analysis of data from the OASIS 5 trial compared the short-term costs and long-term effectiveness of fondaparinux and enoxaparin in 20,078 patients with non-ST-elevation acute coronary syndromes. The original trial had shown that fondaparinux approximately halved the rate of major bleeding at 9 days compared with enoxaparin after randomisation, and clinical outcomes at 6 months were comparable between the two regimens. A 180-day cost analysis revealed that fondaparinux would result in a cost saving of US$546 per patient versus enoxaparin, with savings varying between US$494 and US$733. Of the total difference in costs, 80% was accounted for by the short-term clinical benefits of fondaparinux, excluding the acquisition cost difference. Over the long term, fondaparinux was predicted to generate a US$188 saving and 0.04 additional QALYs in the average patient over enoxaparin, with the dominance of fondaparinux maintained in both low- and high-risk patients [7].

Therefore, while the use of thromboprophylaxis is associated with higher medical costs than the absence of thromboprophylaxis, it represents a cost-effective use of healthcare resources in acutely ill medical inpatients [1].

References

1. Griffin J. Deep vein thrombosis and pulmonary embolism. London: Office of Health Economics; 1996.
2. Bergqvist D, Jendteg S, Johansen L, et al. Cost of long-term complications of deep venous thrombosis of the lower extremities: an analysis of a defined patient population in Sweden. Ann Intern Med 1997; 126:454–457.
3. Pechevis, M, Detournay B, Pribil C, et al. Economic evaluation of enoxaparin vs. placebo for the prevention of venous thromboembolism in acutely ill medical patients. Value Health 2000; 3:389–396.
4. Lloyd AC, Anderson PM, Quinlan DJ, et al. Economic evaluation of the use of enoxaparin for thromboprophylaxis in acutely ill medical patients. J Med Econ 2001; 4:99–113.
5. de Lissovoy G, Subedi P. Economic evaluation of enoxaparin as prophylaxis against venous thromboembolism in seriously ill medical patients: a US perspective. Am J Manag Care 2002; 8:1082–1088.
6. McGarry LJ, Thompson D, Weinstein MC, et al. Cost effectiveness of thromboprophylaxis with a low-molecular-weight heparin versus unfractionated heparin in acutely ill medical inpatients. Am J Manag Care 2004; 10:632–642.
7. Sculpher MJ, Lozano-Ortega G, Sambrook J, et al. Fondaparinux versus enoxaparin in non-ST-elevation acute coronary syndromes: Short-term costs and long-term cost-effectiveness using data from the Fifth Organization to Assess Strategies in Acute Ischemic Syndromes Investigators (OASIS-5) trial. Am Heart J 2009; 157: 845–852.

Chapter 4

Introduction to thromboprophylaxis in surgical patients

Achieving a balance

The thromboembolism risk associated with surgery varies according to the procedure being performed, with some surgical procedures carrying little or no risk and others carrying a very high risk. Thromboprophylaxis is effective but is associated with expense, inconvenience and adverse effects. Therefore, it is necessary to make a balanced judgement for each patient. Three key aspects must be considered:

- patient risk;
- procedure risk; and
- prophylactic method – efficacy, safety, cost and convenience.

When considering prophylaxis for surgical patients, there are two general approaches. In the first approach, the risk of VTE is estimated by summating the individual's predisposing factors (Figure 4.1) and the risk of surgical procedures (Figure 4.2) [1]. Data on the risk of clinical thromboembolism (thrombophlebitis, nonfatal PE, fatal PE and chronic venous change) are sparse; the risk is usually assumed from studies using venography as a surrogate (Figure 4.2) [2].

The next step is to balance the efficacy of a prophylactic method against safety, cost and convenience. Prophylactic methods can be broadly divided into mechanical and pharmacological methods; each has relative advantages and disadvantages, which are empirically summarised in Figure 4.3. Most of the data are derived from orthopaedic studies, but the principles can be reasonably extrapolated to other surgical procedures. In the other approach, prophylaxis is routinely implemented to all patients belonging to each of the major target groups, such as those undergoing major general surgery or major orthopaedic surgery [1].

Individual risk factors for surgical patients

Previous or personal history of VTE
Increasing age (>60 years at particular risk)
Prolonged immobility (>4 weeks before or after surgery)
Recent myocardial infarction or stroke (paralysis)
Central venous catheter in situ
Cancer (including treatment)
Obesity (BMI ≥30 kg/m^2)
Varicose veins with associated phlebitis
Severe infection
Inflammatory bowel disease
Dehydration
Known thrombophilias
Use of HRT / oestrogen-containing hormonal contraception

Figure 4.1 BMI, body mass index; HRT, hormone replacement therapy; VTE, venous thromboembolism. Adapted from NICE [3].

Surgical procedures and risk

Procedure	Venographic DVT (%)	Symptomatic DVT (%)	Fatal PE (%)
Hip replacement	60	4	0.4
Knee replacement	65	4–10	0.2
Hip fracture	60	4	2?
Polytrauma	55	?	?
Cancer surgery	30	?	??
Spinal surgery	35	?	?
Major gynaecological surgery	20	–	–

Figure 4.2 DVT, deep vein thrombosis; PE, pulmonary embolism. Adapted from Nicolaides et al. [2].

Currently available prophylaxis in surgery

Method	Efficacy	Safety	Convenience	Cost
Mechanical				
Stockings	+	+++	++	£
Foot pumps	++	+++	+	£££
IPC	+++	+++	+	£££
Pharmacological				
Warfarin	++	+	+	££
LMWH	+++	++	++	££
Pentasaccharide	+++/++++	+	+++	£££
Aspirin	+/−	+	++++	£
Unfractionated heparin	++	+	++	££
Oral anti-Xa/Anti- thrombin	+++	++	+++	££

Figure 4.3 IPC, intermittent pneumatic compression; LMWH, low-molecular-weight heparin.

Guidelines

It is wise for each surgical department to combine common sense and experience with evidence to produce guidelines for thromboprophylaxis. These guidelines should ensure the routine and automatic provision of prophylaxis, yet allow flexibility when required by individual patient circumstances. This should give the patient the benefit of best practice and give the hospital protection against risk [4].

NICE recommends mechanical prophylaxis for all surgical patients, regardless of the type of procedure being performed, which means that all patients should receive compression/anti-embolism stockings, intermittent pneumatic compression devices and/or foot impulse devices [3]. For high-risk patients or those with additional risk factors, additional anticoagulation with LMWH or fondaparinux is advised (Figure 4.4) [3]. The DoH Working Group on Venous Thromboembolism reported that low-risk surgical patients need early mobilisation and that thromboprophylaxis is needed only if patients develop a risk factor that places them at intermediate or higher risk. Aspirin is not recommended as a form of thromboprophylaxis [5].

However, the Royal College of Obstetricians and Gynaecologists (RCOG) has raised concern over the NICE recommendations, stating that the risk categories need to be re-evaluated and that there is limited evidence for the use of mechanical prophylaxis or fondaparinux over LMWH [6]. The RCOG states that medical conditions, such as heart failure, are not included and that patients over 40 years rather than 60 years should be considered to be at particular risk of VTE and therefore be candidates for anticoagulant therapy.

Summary of NICE guidance on thromboprophylaxis in surgical patients	
Thromboprophylaxis type	Patient type (excluding day cases)
Mechanical (GCS, IPC, foot impulse devices)	All surgical patients
LMWH	Gynaecological, cardiac*, thoracic, urological, neurosurgical†, vascular if one or more patient-related risk factors present, otherwise mechanical alone
LMWH or fondaparinux	Elective hip replacement, hip fracture‡, knee replacement, continue for 4 weeks if one or more patient-related risk factor

Figure 4.4 GCS, graduated compression stockings; IPC, intermittent pneumatic compression. *If no other anticoagulant is being used. †Excepting unsecured lesions (ruptured cranial or spinal vascular malformations). ‡Continue for 4 weeks even if no patient-related risk factors present. Adapted from NICE [3].

References

1. Geerts WH, Berqvist D, Pineo GF, et al. Prevention of venous thromboembolism. American College of Chest Physicians Evidence-Based Clinical Practice Guidelines. Chest 2008; 133(6, Suppl):381S–453S.

2. Nicolaides AN, Breddin HK, Fareed J, et al. Prevention and treatment of venous thromboembolism. International Consensus Statement (guidelines according to scientific evidence). Int Angiol. 2006; 25:101–161.

3. National Institute of Clinical Excellence. Venous thromboembolism - reducing the risk NICE clinical guidelines CG92 (January 2010). Available at: www.nice.org.uk/nicemedia/pdf/CG92NICEGuidance.pdf.

4. Warwick D, Dahl OE, Fisher WD. Orthopaedic thromboprophylaxis: limitations of current guidelines. J Bone Joint Surg Br 2008; 90-B:127–132.

5. Department of Health. Report of the independent expert working group on the prevention of venous thromboembolism in hospitalised patients. Smart No. 278330 (April 2007). Available at: www.dh.gov.uk/en/Publicationsandstatistics/Publications/PublicationsPolicyAndGuidance/DH_073944.

6. RCOG. Response to NICE VTE guideline consultation (December 2006). Available at: www.rcog.org.uk/resources/Public/pdf/vte_consultation_response.pdf.

Chapter 5

Thromboprophylaxis in orthopaedic surgery

The risk in orthopaedic surgery

Some orthopaedic procedures probably carry no risk of thrombosis (e.g. upper limb surgery), whereas others carry a particularly high risk (e.g. revision hip surgery). Total hip replacement, total knee replacement and hip fracture have been the most widely studied procedures. The rate of fatal PE, without prophylaxis, is around 0.4% for total hip replacement and total knee replacement, and is probably higher for hip fracture. The symptomatic DVT rate for total hip replacement is around 4%. It may be higher for total knee replacement, although the similarity between postoperative and thrombotic swelling or calf pain confounds diagnosis. The frequency of chronic venous insufficiency, an important longer-term outcome, is unknown but is likely to be raised in those with asymptomatic DVT.

The *ACCP 8th Conference on Antithrombotic and Thrombolytic Therapy* recommendations for the prevention of VTE are provided in Figure 5.1 [1]. NICE recommends that, in additional to mechanical methods being offered, all orthopaedic patients undergoing lower-limb surgical procedures or wearing plaster casts should have a risk assessment. Those with risk factors should be offered mechanical prophylaxis and LMWHs, continued until the risk has expired. All those having a knee or hip replacement should be given mechanical thromboprophylaxis and then post operative LMWHs, fondaparinux, dabigatran or rivaroxaban. These should be continued for 2 weeks after knee replacement and 4 to 5 weeks after hip replacement [2].

Mechanical prophylaxis

Because bleeding is of concern to surgeons and anaesthetists, mechanical methods are enticing. GCS are widely used. The stockings should be carefully woven, fit well and must remain in place. There are few data on the efficacy after orthopaedic surgery, but a meta-analysis of studies from elsewhere in surgery suggests that they have a modest benefit. IPC devices (above or below

ACCP consensus conference recommendations						
Procedure	LMWH	Fondaparinux	VFP	VKA	IPC/VFP	Aspirin
THR	1A	1A	NR	1A	1A	NR
TKR	1A	1A	NR	1A	1B	NR
Hip fracture	1B	1A	1C+	1B	1A	NR
Arthroscopy	1B only if risk factors	NR	NR	NR	NR	NR
Spine surgery	1B only if risk factors	NR		NR	NR	1B only if risk factors	NR
Isolated limb trauma	NR	NR	NR	NR	NR	NR
Major trauma	1A	NR	NR	NR	1B	NR

Figure 5.1 The grading system used by the American College of Chest Physicians (ACCP) is defined in Figure 5.2. IPC, intermittent pneumatic compression; LMWH, low-molecular-weight heparin; NR, not recommended; THR, total hip replacement; TKR, total knee replacement; VFP, venous foot pump; VKA, vitamin K antagonist. Based on Geerts et al. [1].

the knee) are effective, particularly after knee surgery. Foot pumps rhythmically empty the plantar venous plexus of the foot, flushing out the deep leg veins, offering prophylaxis that is probably equivalent to LMWH. They work best without the simultaneous use of graduated stockings and with the leg flat or slightly hanging down to enhance the preload required to prime the foot plexus.

Compliance and expense are issues for all mechanical methods; they are not suitable for, nor is there evidence in favour of, extended duration prophylaxis with mechanical devices.

Pharmacological methods
Warfarin
Warfarin is still widely used in North America. Death from PE in patients taking warfarin is exceedingly rare; the drug is nearly as effective as LMWH in reducing venographic DVT. It is supported by the main consensus groups and can be delivered beyond hospital discharge to protect against the risk of late-onset VTE. It is, however, regarded as obsolete in much of Europe because of the narrow window of safety, the need for regular coagulation monitoring, the delayed lead-time to effect, and the potential interaction with drugs or alcohol. It may not be as safe and efficacious in real clinical practice as it is in

a well-controlled clinical trial. The *ACCP 8th Conference on Antithrombotic and Thrombolytic Therapy* recommended that for patients undergoing elective total hip replacement or knee athroscopy, warfarin should be used to ensure a target international normalised ratio (INR) of 2.5 (range 2.0–3.0) [1]. This Grade 1A recommendation (see Figure 5.2) is also supported by a recommendation that such thromboprophylaxis should continue for a minimum of 10 days in patients undergoing hip or knee arthroplasty or hip fracture surgery (Grade 1A), and that it should continue for over 10 and up to 35 days in patients having hip arthroplasty or hip fracture surgery (Grade 1A) [1]. NICE states that oral anticoagulants such as warfarin are less effective than UFH or LMWH and significantly increase the risk of bleeding [2].

Fondaparinux

Fondaparinux is a synthetic pentasaccharide that specifically inhibits factor Xa. It has a 100% bioavailability, is not metabolised and is renally excreted. The half-life is 15 hours, allowing once-daily administration. Fondaparinux has been compared with the LMWH enoxaparin in over 7300 hip replacement, knee replacement and hip fracture patients. The overall VTE rate at 11 days after surgery (venographic DVT plus symptomatic DVT or PE) was reduced from 13.7% with enoxaparin to 6.8% with fondaparinux (odds reduction 55.2%; 95% confidence interval [CI] 45.8–63.1, $p<0.001$) [4]. Some of this advantage in VTE (and disadvantage in bleeding) may be explained by a different timing schedule than used with LMWH, as fondaparinux was given in closer proximity to surgery [5]. Furthermore, the apparent advantage of fondaparinux was established for asymptomatic event rates rather than for symptomatic rates. In the international, multicentre, nonrandomised, open-label, prospective, intervention EXPERT trial, 5704 patients undergoing major orthopaedic surgery of the lower limb were given a daily subcutaneous injection of 2.5 mg fondaparinux for

American College of Chest Physicians grades of evidence	
Number grades	
1	Clear risk–benefit ratio
2	Unclear risk–benefit ratio
Letter grades	
A	RCTs without important limitations and with consistent results
B	RCTs with important limitations (i.e. inconsistent results or methodological flaws)
C+	No RCTs but expert opinion that strong RCT results can be extrapolated, or overwhelming evidence from observational studies
C	Observational studies or extrapolation from other trials

Figure 5.2 RCT, randomised controlled trial [3].

3–5 weeks postoperatively, of whom 1631 had a neuroaxial or deep peripheral nerve catheter. The last fondaparinux dose was given 36 hours before catheter removal, with the next dose administered 12 hours after catheter removal. The rate of symptomatic VTE at 4–6 weeks after surgery was 0.8% in catheter patients and 1.1% in patients without a catheter, which was below the predetermined margin of noninferiority, while the overall rate of major bleeding was 0.8%, with no significant differences between patients with and without a catheter. Consequently, fondaparinux was shown to be safe and effective not only after major orthopaedic lower limb surgery but also when the drug is disontinued for 48 hours to allow catheter removal [6]. The drug is not readily reversed and is contraindicated in renal impairment. NICE states that fondaparinux may be used as an alternative to LMWHs within its licensed indications [2]. However, the RCOG notes that data on fondaparinux are not as extensive as that on LMWHs, and while it is useful to include this agent in the guidelines, it may be associated with more bleeding events that LMWHs or UFHs [7].

Aspirin
Aspirin is superficially attractive as it is familiar and cheap. However, the Pulmonary Embolism Prevention (PEP) study examined over 17,000 hip fracture and arthroplasty patients randomly allocated to placebo or aspirin [8]. The death rate was identical in each group. The risk reduction for DVT and PE (in a post-hoc analysis) was only approximately 30% (50% less than is expected from LMWH); the reduction in symptomatic VTE was matched by an increase in bleeding events. Because the weak effect on VTE was annulled by adverse effects, it is not to be recommended [1,9].

Low-molecular-weight heparins
LMWH is the most widely studied class of thromboprophylactic agents in orthopaedics. LMWH can be administered once (Europe) or twice daily (North America), and no monitoring is required. LMWH is superior to dextran and UFH and at least as effective as warfarin and mechanical pumps. Used carefully, significant bleeding complications are rare. Trials consistently show a risk reduction of around 60% compared with control in major trauma, hip and knee replacement, and hip fracture. There are also data to support its use in selected patients with knee arthroscopy or plaster casts.

The ACCP guidelines recommend that LMWHs are given for over 10 days in hip or knee arthroplasty or hip fracture surgery (Grade 1A), and for over 10 days and up to 35 days in hip athroplasty and hip fracture surgery (Grade 1A) [1]. NICE also recommends prolonged (28–35 days) LMWH therapy in patients undergoing hip fracture surgery and in those undergoing other orthopaedic procedures if they have other risk factors for VTE [2].

Direct anti-Xa inhibitors and direct thrombin IIa inhibitors

These drugs were licensed for use in 2008 and will transform thromboprophylaxis. They are administered orally and have a broad therapeutic and safety window; therefore, monitoring is not required. Unlike LMWHs and fondaparinux they avoid the need for regular injections, which can be troublesome in extended out-of-hospital prophylaxis for some patients after joint replacement, hip fracture, major trauma, spinal injury or patients in plaster casts. They also avoid the complex monitoring that is required for warfarin. The first dose is given after surgery and the medication can be continued for as long as the patient is at risk of VTE. The drugs are difficult to reverse. Presently, two are available: a direct thrombin inhibitor, dabigatran, and an anti-Xa inhibitor, rivaroxaban, both of which have been recommended by NICE as an option for the prevention of venous thromboembolism in adults having elective total hip replacement or elective total knee replacement surgery [10,11].

For dabigatran, the onset and offset of anticoagulant activity are rapid and predictable. It is recommended that treatment is initiated 1–4 hours after surgery, with only half a dose on the day after surgery. Dabigatran can be given once daily, with the 150-mg dose for use in patients aged ≥75 years and in those with moderate renal impairment, and the 220-mg dose in all other patients. Studies have indicated that dabigatran achieves comparable outcomes to enoxaparin, with similar efficacy and a similar safety profile [12]. In the RE-MODEL randomized, double-blind trial, in which dabigatran 150 mg or 220 mg once daily was compared with subcutaneous enoxaparin 40 mg once daily in 1076 patients undergoing total knee replacement who were treated for 6–10 days and followed-up for 3 months, both doses of dabigatran were noninferior to enoxaparin on the combined end point of total VTE and mortality during treatment, and there was no significant difference in the incidence of bleeding events [13]. In the double-blind, randomized RE-NOVATE trial, dabigatran 150 mg or 220 mg once daily was compared with subcutaneous enoxaparin 40 mg once daily for 28–35 days in 3494 patients undergoing total hip replacement. Again, both dabigatran doses were non-inferior to enoxaparin for the combined end point of total VTE and death during treatment, and there was no significant difference in major bleeding rates [14]. Both studies also demonstrated that there were no differences between dabigatran and enoxaparin groups in terms of increases in liver enzyme concentrations and the incidence of acute coronary events [13,14].

Phase II studies of rivaroxaban have demonstrated safety and efficacy for thromboprophylaxis after total hip or total knee replacement surgery, with a wide therapeutic window [12]. A pooled analysis of four studies of rivaroxaban for the prevention of VTE after orthopaedic surgery, in which a total of 12,729 patients were randomised to oral rivaroxaban 10 mg once daily starting 6–8 hours after surgery or subcutaneous enoxaparin 40 mg once daily or 30 mg twice daily, showed that rivarobaxan significantly reduced the incidence of symptomatic VTE and death compared with enoxaparin regimens at day 12 and for the total duration of the studies [13]. There was no significant increase in the risk of major bleeding with rivaroxaban [13]. Another phase II trial (ATLAS ACT-TIMI-46) of rivaroxaban or placebo administered to 3491 recent acute coronary syndrome patients also treated with aspirin or aspirin plus clopidogrel indicated that best doses to test in a phase III study would be 2.5 mg and 5.0 mg twice daily [15]. In addition, rivarobaxan was shown to significantly reduce the incidence of the combined end point of death, myocardial infarction, and stroke compared with placebo, at an absolute risk reduction of 1.6% [15].

Particular aspects of low-molecular-weight heparin thromboprophylaxis

Proximity of dosing and surgery

The closer to surgery that pharmacological prophylaxis is administered, the better the thromboprophylaxis is, but this also correlates with an increased risk of bleeding. In Europe, LMWHs are given prior to surgery (e.g. enoxaparin 40 mg once daily starting 12 hours pre-operatively), presumably so there is an anticoagulant effect to counteract the thrombogenic factors during surgery (tissue thromboplastins and venous stasis). However, if the drug is given too long before surgery, plasma levels will be too low for any prophylactic effect; if given too close to surgery then surgical bleeding can be expected [16]. In North America, LMWHs are given after surgery at a higher dose and more frequently (e.g. enoxaparin 30 mg twice daily). This may reduce the risk of surgical bleeding, but the intra-operative risk factors are not covered and thrombi may have begun to form during sugery [17]. The drug is now expected to be therapeutic rather than prophylactic. Prophylaxis with pharmacological agents, such as LMWHs and pentasaccharides, needs to be given close but not too close, to surgery. In the UK and Europe, patients receiving 40 mg enoxaparin may receive it 12 hours prior to surgery [2] although the NICE guidelines recommend post-operative administration to ensure a proper interval from the surgical procedure.

Neuraxial anaesthesia

Orthopaedic patients will benefit from neuraxial (i.e. spinal or epidural) anaesthesia (reduced mortality, enhanced analgesia, weak thromboprophylactic effect). Initial European experience with LMWHs reassured that neuraxial anaesthesia could be safely used in their presence, but the US FDA has raised concerns that spinal haematomata may occur. It is prudent not to use neuraxial anaesthesia and LMWHs within 12 hours of each other and to ensure such patients are not receiving other drugs – for example, nonsteroidal anti-inflammatory drugs – that might interfere with coagulation and, therefore, increase the risk of bleeding. The interval for pentasaccharides (e.g. fondaparinux), with their longer half-lives, is likely to be longer [18,19].

Extended-duration prophylaxis

Earlier LMWH studies established that prophylaxis for 7–10 days (while the patient was in hospital) would reduce the venographic DVT rate by 60%. However, consistent evidence from several sources shows that half of symptomatic thromboses after knee replacement and two-thirds after hip replacement occur beyond the second week, usually when the patient has been discharged from hospital [20]. Several recent randomised trials have proven that the risk of thrombosis after hospital discharge in hip surgery can be reduced by two-thirds if LMWH is continued for at least 4 weeks. The advantage for extended prophylaxis in knee replacement is not so clear [21].

A meta-analysis by Eikelboom et al. shows that extending the duration of LMWH for approximately 5 weeks after hip replacement will reduce the venographic DVT rate from 21% to 8.2% [21]. These studies were large enough to show that the frequency of symptomatic VTE was reduced by the same proportion, from 4.5% to 1.7% (risk reduction 62%). Therefore, it can now be shown with confidence that venographic surrogates do reflect clinical reality – until these extended duration studies, this was only an assumption [22].

These studies show that the number to treat to prevent one symptomatic DVT or PE after hip replacement is 37; from this figure, the cost effectiveness can be calculated. Because the cost of LMWH is relatively low, and the cost of investigation or treatment of thromboembolism is relatively high, this is likely to be a cost-effective approach [23,24].

Discharge at 4 days after joint replacement surgery is common and minimally invasive, and day-case hip surgery is being designed. Therefore, systems need to be considered for administering and financing thromboprophylaxis after hospital discharge. The new oral agents will offer a pragmatic solution to the administration of extended-duration prophylaxis.

Recommendations for specific orthopaedic procedures

Knee arthroscopy

Symptomatic VTE without prophylaxis is very rare – less than 1%, although venographic DVT frequencies from around 3% to as high as 18% have been reported. Prophylaxis with LMWHs probably reduces the risk without major bleeding complications [25–30]. The ACCP and NICE guidelines recommend that LMWH prophylaxis is given to those undergoing knee arthroscopy if additional risk factors are present and if the surgery is complicated [1,2].

Trauma

Polytrauma patients

With thromboplastin release, major surgical interventions and subsequent prolonged immobility patients with multiple trauma are at particularly high risk of VTE. Systematic venography has shown a DVT frequency of 58% in these patients. Prophylaxis with LMWHs is likely to reduce the frequency of VTE but is contraindicated in associated head injury, spinal injury, visceral injury and widespread soft tissue injury [31]. Mechanical methods are an attractive alternative, although these devices have practical limitations because concomitant lower limb injuries may preclude their application; the evidence base is limited to a few small studies [32].

Isolated lower limb trauma

Due to this group's extensive heterogeneity and limited evidence base, clear recommendations cannot be devised. Routine prophylaxis for isolated lower limb trauma cannot be substantiated by present data; however the ACCP, NICE and others recommend a thorough risk assessment and an approach standardised within an institution, yet individualised to each injured patient, [1,2,33–40].

Spinal surgery

Spinal surgery carries a risk of VTE; however, pharmacological prophylaxis carries a risk of bleeding around the spinal cord. For straightforward cases, the risk–benefit ratio supports no routine prophylaxis except early mobilisation, perhaps potentiated by mechanical methods. For those with greater risk factors for VTE, LMWHs or mechanical methods should be used (although no robust studies have been conducted to support this).

References

1. Geerts WH, Bergqvist D, Pineo GF, et al. Prevention of venous thromboembolism. American College of Chest Physicians Evidence-Based Clinical Practice Guidelines. Chest 2008; 133(6, Suppl):381S–453S.

2. National Institute of Clinical Excellence. Venous thromboembolism – reducing the risk NICE clinical guidelines CG92 (January 2010). Available at: www.nice.org.uk/nicemedia/pdf/CG92NICEGuidance.pdf.

3. Guyatt G, Schünemann HJ, Cook D, et al. Applying the grades of recommendation for antithrombotic and thrombolytic therapy: the Seventh ACCP Conference on Antithrombotic and Thrombolytic Therapy. Chest. 2004; 126(Suppl):179S–187S.

4. Turpie AGG, Bauer KA, Eriksson BI, et al. Fondaparinux vs enoxaparin for the prevention of venous thromboembolism in major orthopaedic surgery. Arch Int Med 2002; 162:1833–1840.

5. Lowe GD, Sandercock PA, Rosendaal FR. Prevention of venous thromboembolism after major orthopaedic surgery: is fondaparinux an advance? Lancet 2003; 362:504–505.

6. Singelyn FJ, Verheyen CCPM, Piovella F, et al. The safety and efficacy of extended thromboprophylaxis with fondaparinux after major orthopedic surgery of the lower limb with or without a neuraxial or deep peripheral nerve catheter: The EXPERT study. Anesth Analg 2007; 105:1540–1547.

7. RCOG. Response to NICE VTE guideline consultation (December 2006). Available at: www.rcog.org.uk/resources/Public/pdf/vte_consultation_response.pdf.

8. Prevention of pulmonary embolism and deep vein thrombosis with low dose aspirin: Pulmonary Embolism Prevention (PEP) trial. Lancet 2000; 355:1295–1302.

9. Cohen A, Quinlan D. PEP trial. Pulmonary Embolism Prevention. Lancet 2000; 356:247.

10. National Institute for Health and Clinical Excellence. NICE technology appraisal guidance 157. Dabigatran etexilate for the prevention of venous thromboembolism after hip or knee replacement surgery in adults. London: NICE, 2008.

11. National Institute for Health and Clinical Excellence. NICE technology appraisal guidance 170. Rivaroxaban for the prevention of venous thromboembolism after hip or knee replacement in adults. London: NICE, 2009.

12. Rosencher N, Bellamy L, Arnaout L. Should new oral anticoagulants replace low-molecular-weight heparin for thromboprophylaxis in orthopaedic surgery? Arch Cardiovasc Dis 2009; 102:327–333.

13. Eriksson BI, Dahl OE, Rosencher N, et al. Oral dabigatran etexilate vs. subcutaneous enoxaparin for the prevention of venous thromboembolism after total knee replacement: the RE-MODEL randomized trial. J Thromb Haemost 2007; 5:2178–2185.

14. Eriksson BI, Dahl OE, Rosencher N, et al. Dabigatran etexilate versus enoxaparin for prevention of venous thromboembolism after total hip replacement: a randomised, double-blind, non-inferiority trial. Lancet 2007; 370:949–956.

15. Mega JL, Braunwald E, Mohanavelu S, et al; on behalf of the ATLAS ACS-TIMI 46 study group. Rivaroxaban versus placebo in patients with acute coronary syndromes (ATLAS ACS-TIMI 46): a randomised, double-blind, phase II trial. Lancet 2009; 374: 29–38.

16. Hull RD, Pineo GF, Stein PD, et al. Timing of initial administration of low-molecular-weight heparin prophylaxis against deep vein thrombosis in patients following elective hip arthroplasty: a systematic review. Arch Intern Med 2001; 161:1952–1960.

17. Strebel N, Prins M, Agnelli G, et al. Preoperative or postoperative start of prophylaxis for S venous thromboembolism with low-molecular-weight heparin in elective hip surgery? Arch Intern Med 2002; 162:1451–1456.

18. Horlocker TT. Low molecular weight heparin and neuraxial anesthesia. Thromb Res 2001; 101:141–154.

19. Bergqvist D, Lindblad B, Matsch T. Low molecular weight heparin for thromboprophylaxis and epidural/regional anaesthesia – is there a risk? Acta Anaesthesiol Scand 1992; 36:605–609.

20. Warwick D, Friedman RJ, Agnelli G, et al. Insufficient duration of venous thromboembolism prophylaxis after total hip or knee replacement when compared with the time course of thromboembolic events: Findings from the GLORY Global Orthopaedic Registry. J Bone Joint Surg Br 2007; 89-B:799–807.
21. Eikelboom JW, Quinlan DJ, Douketis JD. Extended-duration prophylaxis against venous thromboembolism after total hip or knee replacement: a meta-analysis of the randomised trials. Lancet 2001; 358:9–15.
22. Dahl OE, Gudmundsen TE, Haukeland L. Late occurring clinical deep vein thrombosis in joint-operated patients. Acta Orthop Scand 2000; 71:47–50.
23. Cohen A, Bailey CS, Alikhan R, et al. Extended thromboprophylaxis with low molecular weight heparin reduces symptomatic venous thromboembolism following lower limb arthroplasty. Thromb Haemost 2001; 85:940–941.
24. Friedman RJ, Dunsworth GA. Cost analysis of extended prophylaxis with enoxaparin after hip arthroplasty. Clin Orthop Relat Res 2000; 370:171–182.
25. Demers C, Marcoux S, Ginsberg JS, et al. Incidence of venographically proved deep vein thrombosis after knee arthroscopy. Arch Intern Med 1998; 158:47–50.
26. Durica S, Raskob G, Johnson C, et al. Incidence of deep-vein thrombosis after arthroscopic knee surgery. Thromb Haemost 1997; 77(Suppl):183.
27. Jaureguito JW, Greenwald AE, Wilcox JF, et al. The incidence of deep venous thrombosis after arthroscopic knee surgery. Am J Sports Med 1999; 27:707–710.
28. Michot M, Conen D, Holtz D, et al. Prevention of deep-vein thrombosis in ambulatory arthroscopic knee surgery: a randomized trial of prophylaxis with low-molecular weight heparin. Arthroscopy 2002; 18:257–263.
29. Schippinger G, Wirnsberger GH, Obernosterer A, et al. Thromboembolic complications after arthroscopic knee surgery; Incidence and risk factors in 101 patients. Acta Orthop Scand 1998; 68:144–146.
30. Wirth T, Schneider B, Misselwitz F, et al. Prevention of venous thromboembolism after knee arthroscopy with low-molecular weight heparin (reviparin): results of a randomized controlled trial. Arthroscopy 2001; 17:393–399.
31. Geerts WH, Jay RM, Code KI, et al. A comparison of low-dose heparin with low-molecular-weight heparin as prophylaxis against venous thromboembolism after major trauma. N Engl J Med 1996; 335:701–707.
32. Knudson MM, Morabito D, Paiement GD, et al. Use of low molecular weight heparin in preventing thromboembolism in trauma patients. J Trauma 1996; 41:446–459.
33. Abelseth G, Buckley RE, Pineo GE, et al. Incidence of deep-vein thrombosis in patients with fractures of the lower extremity distal to the hip. J Orthop Trauma 1996; 10:230–235.
34. Elliott CG, Dudney TM, Egger M, et al. Calf-thigh sequential pneumatic compression compared with plantar venous pneumatic compression to prevent deep-vein thrombosis after non-lower extremity trauma. J Trauma 1999; 47:25–32.
35. Fisher CG, Blachut PA, Salvian AJ, et al. Effectiveness of pneumatic leg compression devices for the prevention of thromboembolic disease in orthopaedic trauma patients: a prospective, randomized study of compression alone versus no prophylaxis. J Orthop Trauma 1995; 9:1–7.
36. Jørgensen PS, Warming T, Hansen K, et al. Low molecular weight heparin (Innohep) as thromboprophylaxis in outpatients with a plaster cast: a venografic controlled study. Thromb Res 2002; 105:477–480.
37. Kock H-J, Schmit-Neuerburg KP, Hanke J, et al. Thromboprophylaxis with low-molecular-weight heparin in outpatients with plaster-cast immobilisation of the leg. Lancet 1995; 346:459–461.
38. Kujath P, Spannagel U, Habscheid W. Incidence and prophylaxis of deep venous thrombosis in outpatients with injury of the lower limb. Haemostasis 1993; 3(Suppl 1):20–26.

39. Lassen MR, Borris LC, Nakov RL. Use of the low-molecular-weight heparin reviparin to prevent deep-vein thrombosis after leg injury requiring immobilization. N Engl J Med 2002; 347:726–730; correspondence 2003; 348:1062.
40. Spannagel U, Kujath P. Low molecular weight heparin for the prevention of thromboembolism in outpatients immobilized by plaster cast. Semin Thromb Hemost 1993; 19(Suppl 1):131–141.

Chapter 6

Thromboprophylaxis in cancer surgery

The presence of cancer, overt or occult, is thrombogenic to the individual. This has been recognised from the time of Armand Trousseau who, in 1865 [1], stated: "I have long been struck with the frequency with which cancerous patients are affected with painful oedema of the superior or inferior extremities, whether or not either was the seat of the cancer. The frequent occurrence of *phlegmasia alba dolens* with an appreciable cancerous tumour, led me to the inquiry of whether a relationship of cause and effect did not exist between the two". This observation is classically associated with pancreatic carcinoma but other tumours, particularly adenocarcinomas, can also cause it. Trousseau correctly diagnosed it in himself scarcely 18 months later and died of stomach cancer in 1867 [2].

Pathophysiology

Mucinous adenocarcinomas secrete abnormally glycosylated mucins and mucin fragments into the bloodstream [3]. Such tumours, grown in tissue culture, produce a supernatant that is tumour-free but characteristically shows marked thrombogenic properties. It is this secretion of abnormal mucins that leads to the hypercoagulable state in some malignancies and the association with VTE. There are many reported abnormalities within the coagulation pathways but these are inconsistent between types of cancer. Some individuals have a shortening of the activated partial thromboplastin time; in others, a reduction in levels of protein C or antithrombin are reported. Platelet activation can, occasionally, be seen together with activation of inflammatory pathways. Recent evidence has shown that tumour-induced coagulation activation is intrinsically involved with tumour cell growth, angiogenesis and metastasis. Continuous treatment with heparin is usually required to prevent recurrent episodes of thrombosis, but oral anticoagulants (vitamin K antagonists) that also decrease thrombin production are often ineffective [4–6].

Epidemiology

VTE is a common complication in cancer patients and an important cause of morbidity and mortality. The development of VTE in the cancer patient is associated with a reduced prognosis. Malignancy alone increases the risk of VTE fourfold and this is increased to between six and seven times the normal risk when chemotherapy is introduced as a treatment [7]. One in seven hospitalised cancer patients who die do so from a PE [8]. Of these patients, 60% have a localised cancer or limited metastatic disease, which would have otherwise allowed for a reasonably long survival in the absence of the fatal embolic event.

Venography is the usual method of detection of venous thrombosis in clinical trials. However, the clinical relevance of venographically detected DVT is unclear and the prevalence of this complication in clinical trials is not necessarily representative of the overall cancer surgery clinical risk. @RISTOS was a prospective registry of consecutive patients undergoing gynaecological or urological cancer surgery [9]. From November 2000 to October 2001, 2373 patients were included in the study in 31 Italian hospitals: 52% undergoing general surgery, 29% urological surgery and 19% gynaecological surgery. A follow-up, as scheduled by study protocol, was obtained in 99.5% of patients. In-hospital prophylaxis was performed in 81.6% and post-discharge prophylaxis in 30.7% of the patients. The study found:

- The overall death rate was 1.72% and nearly half of these cases were due to VTE.
- A total of 50 patients (2.1%) were found to be affected by clinically overt VTE by the adjudication committee (DVT 0.42%, nonfatal PE 0.88% and death 0.80%).
- The incidence of VTE was 2.83% in general surgery, 2.0% in gynaecological surgery and 0.87% in urological surgery.
- Of the events, 40% occurred more than 21 days after surgery.
- Five risk factors were identified: age greater than 60 years, previous VTE, advanced cancer, duration of anaesthesia greater than 2 hours and bed resting for more than 3 days.

Antithrombotic agents in cancer thromboprophylaxis

The advent of LMWHs in the late 1980s and their apparent safety profile provided a further agent in the armamentarium for thromboprophylaxis. It soon became clear that LMWHs (initially in combination with DHE) were at least as effective as low-dose UFHs [10] with a lesser incidence of bleeding and ease of administration, particularly as the newer LMWHs could be administered once daily. A recent review of the LMWHs has demonstrated that, as a group, these agents are an effective and safe alternative to UFHs [11].

Two studies have compared the use of LMWHs and UFHs in patients undergoing craniotomy for malignant brain tumours [12,13]. All patients also received pneumatic compression devices as well as compression stockings. Both studies concluded that both heparin regimens were effective and safe and were associated with a low incidence of VTE when used in combination with intermittent pneumatic devices.

The ENOXAparin in CANcer (ENOXACAN) study group [14] examined patients undergoing surgery for malignant disease and investigated the efficacy of enoxaparin 40 mg once daily beginning before surgery in comparison with low-dose UFH. The study was designed as a prospective, double-blind, randomised, multicentre trial with participating departments from ten countries. The primary outcome, VTE, was detected by mandatory bilateral venography and pulmonary scintigraphy. Follow-up was for 3 months. Of the 631 evaluable patients, 104 (16.5%) developed thromboembolic complications. The frequency was 18.2% in the UFH group and 14.7% in the enoxaparin group. There was no difference in the bleeding events or other complications. No difference in mortality at 30 days or 3 months was also detected. In summary, enoxaparin 40 mg once daily was found to be as safe and effective as UFH given three times daily in preventing VTE in patients undergoing major elective surgery for abdominal or pelvic malignancy.

A meta-analysis of 14 randomised controlled trials compared LMWH and UFH for perioperative thromboprophylaxis in a total of 5502 patients undergoing surgery for cancer. There was no significant difference in mortality rates between patients receiving LMWH and those given UFH, at a relative risk of 0.89. There were also no significant differences in the occurrence of clinically suspected DVT, PE, minor bleeding, or major bleeding, at relative risks of 0.73, 0.60, 0.88, and 0.95, respectively. In a post hoc analysis of DVT outcome using any diagnostic strategy, LMWH was superior to UFH twice daily, at a relative risk of 0.66, but not superior to UFH administered three times daily [15].

The clinical approach to cancer thromboprophylaxis

Surgeons' perceptions regarding the risk of thrombosis in cancer patients undergoing surgery have been highlighted in the Fundamental Research in Oncology and Thrombosis (FRONTLINE) survey [16]. This survey of clinical approaches to thrombosis prevention in cancer patients was undertaken in 2001. At that time, just over half of the respondents would routinely use thromboprophylaxis, usually heparin, in cancer surgical patients. About a further 43% would decide on a case-by-case basis. The majority of respondents reported using thromboprophylaxis in cancer surgical patients for the duration of their hospital stay, although 25% would continue treatment only for 5–10 days. Within the UK, a study of the attitudes of general surgeons to thromboprophylaxis produced virtually identical results [17]. Shortly afterwards, the ENOXACAN II study [18] clearly demonstrated that thromboprophylaxis with a LMWH for 4 weeks after surgery for abdominal or pelvic cancer significantly reduced the incidence of thrombosis, compared with treatment for just 1 week post-surgery (VTE 12% in placebo group [20/167], 4.8% in the LMWH group [8/165]; p=0.02) [18].

Recommendations

Cancer surgery is high-risk surgery and there are few recognised recommendations for the management of cancer patients undergoing such surgery. The SIGN guidelines [19] suggest that both UFH and LMWH given subcutaneously are effective in cancer surgery thromboprophylaxis and that this is improved further by the addition of graduated elastic compression stockings (GECS). These are available as both below-knee and above-knee stockings. Studies comparing above-knee and below-knee stockings have been too small to determine whether or not they are equally effective. Hence, current evidence supports the use of above-knee stockings unless contraindicated (e.g. thigh circumference greater than 81 cm, incontinence). The 8th ACCP guidelines recommend that cancer patients undergoing surgical procedures have routine thromboprophylaxis appropriate for the type of surgery (Grade 1A), while cancer patients confined to bed with an acute medical illness should have routine prophylaxis similar to other high-risk patients (Grade 1A) [21]. Routine prophylaxis should not be used in cancer patients with indwelling central venous catheters (Grade 1B), those receiving chemotherapy or hormonal therapy (Grade 1C), or in order to improve survival (Grade 1B) [20]. Interestingly, patients undergoing major gynaecological or major open urological procedures are identified as particularly high-risk and require low-dose UFH two to three times daily. IPC prophylaxis should be considered in high-risk cancer surgery. However, it has been reported recently that such prophylaxis is likely to fail in women undergoing surgery for gynaecological malignancies [21]. Consideration should be given to the prolonged use of heparin thromboprophylaxis (up to 28 days) in patients undergoing major abdominal cancer surgery.

There are several reasons why LMWH is often the preferred antithrombotic agent over UFH:

- Many of the LMWHs can now be given once daily. This frees up nursing time and is more convenient for home use.
- There is a lesser incidence of heparin-associated thrombocytopenia with LMWH than UFH. LMWH is less likely to be associated with antiplatelet antibodies than UFH.

The use of epidural or spinal regional anaesthetic in itself is associated with a reduction in VTE.

However, concerns have been raised about the possibility of spinal haematoma. This appears to have been more of a problem in the USA than in Europe and may be associated with the timing and dosage of LMWH.

References

1. Trousseau A. Lectures on Clinical Medicine, delivered at the Hotel-Dieu, Paris. Edited and translated by P.V. Bazire. London, UK; The New Sydenham Society Publications. 1868; 55:281–332.
2. Aron E. [The 100th anniversary of the death of A. Trousseau.] Presse Med 1967; 75:1429–1430.
3. Wahrenbrock M, Borsig L, Le D, et al. Selectin-mucin interactions as a probable molecular explanation for the association of Trousseau syndrome with mucinous adenocarcinomas. J Clin Invest 2003; 112:853–862.
4. Sack GH Jr, Levin J, Bell WR. Trousseau's syndrome and other manifestations of chronic disseminated coagulopathy in patients with neoplasms: clinical pathophysiologic, and therapeutic features. Medicine (Baltimore) 1977; 56:1–37.
5. Bell WR, Starksen NF, Tong S, et al. Trousseau's syndrome. Devastating coagulopathy in the absence of heparin. Am J Med 1985; 79:423–430.
6. Krauth D, Holden A, Knapic N, et al. Safety and efficacy of long-term oral anticoagulation in cancer patients. Cancer 1987; 59:983–985.
7. Levitan N, Dowlati A, Remick SC, et al. Rates of initial and recurrent thromboembolic disease among patients with malignancy versus those without malignancy. Risk analysis using Medicare claims data. Medicine (Baltimore) 1999; 178:285–291.
8. Shen VS, Pollak EW. Fatal pulmonary embolism in cancer patients: is heparin prophylaxis justified? South Med J 1980; 73:841–843.
9. Agnelli G, Bolis G, Capussotti L, et al. A clinical outcome-based prospective study on venous thromboembolism in cancer surgery: the @RISTOS project. J Thromb Haemostasis 2003; 1(Suppl 1):Abstract OC191.
10. Baumgartner A, Jacot N, Moser G, et al. Prevention of postoperative deep vein thrombosis by one daily injection of low molecular weight heparin and dihydroergotamine. Vasa 1989; 18:152–156.
11. Holzheimer RG. Low-molecular-weight heparin (LMWH) in the treatment of thrombosis. Eur J Med Res 2004; 9:225–239.
12. Goldhaber SZ, Dunn K, Gerhard-Herman M, et al. Low rate of venous thromboembolism after craniotomy for brain tumor using multimodality prophylaxis. Chest 2002; 122:1933–1937.
13. Macdonald RL, Amidei C, Baron J, et al. Randomized, pilot study of intermittent pneumatic compression devices plus dalteparin versus intermittent pneumatic compression devices plus heparin for prevention of venous thromboembolism in patients undergoing craniotomy. Surg Neurol 2003; 59:363–372; discussion 372–374.
14. ENOXACAN Study Group. Efficacy and safety of enoxaparin versus unfractionated heparin for prevention of deep vein thrombosis in elective cancer surgery: a double-blind randomized multicentre trial with venographic assessment. Br J Surg 1997; 84:1099–1103.
15. Ahl EA, Terrenato I, Barba M, et al. Low-molecular-weight heparin versus unfractionated heparin for perioperative thromboprophylaxis in patients with cancer. Arch Intern Med 2008; 168: 1261–1269.
16. Kakkar AK, Levine M, Pinedo HM, et al. Venous thrombosis in cancer patients: insights from the FRONTLINE survey. Oncologist 2003; 8:381–388.
17. Williams EV, Williams RS, Hughes JL, et al. Prevention of venous thromboembolism in Wales: results of a survey among general surgeons. Postgrad Med J 2002; 78:88–91.
18. Bergqvist D, Agnelli G, Cohen AT, et al; ENOXACAN II Investigators. Duration of prophylaxis against venous thromboembolism with enoxaparin after surgery for cancer. N Engl J Med 2002; 346:975–980.
19. Scottish and Collegiate Guideline Network (SIGN). Prophylaxis of Venous Thromboembolism. London, SIGN publication, 2002; no. 62. Available at: www.sign.ac.uk/guidelines.
20. Geerts WH, Berqvist D, Pineo GF, et al. Prevention of venous thromboembolism. American College of Chest Physicians Evidence-Based Clinical Practice Guidelines. Chest 2008; 133(6, Suppl):381S–453S.
21. Clarke-Pearson DL, Dodge RK, Synan I, et al. Venous thromboembolism prophylaxis: patients at high risk to fail intermittent pneumatic compression. Obstet Gynecol 2003; 101:157–163.

Chapter 7

Thromboprophylaxis in other types of surgery

Whereas the evidence base for surgical thromboprophylaxis has centred on elective orthopaedic surgery and subsequently been adopted in cancer surgery there is a good evidence base for the prevention of thromboembolic disease in other surgical specialities. This chapter will present the evidence base for four surgical specialities – neurological, urological, cardiovascular and gynaecological surgery. A common theme is the difference in elective versus emergency thromboprophylaxis.

Neurological surgery

Acute ischaemic stroke is associated with a high incidence of VTE [1] and reflects the thrombogenicity of damaged neurological tissue. Whilst neurosurgeons are acutely aware of the propensity of their surgery to initiate VTE, surgery within the confines of the cranium or spinal column has always presented the dilemma of balancing the risk between the development of thromboembolism and the disastrous complication of compressive haemorrhage. Neurosurgical patients constitute one of the highest risk groups for postoperative thromboembolic complications.

Neurosurgery performed without thromboprophylaxis produces an incidence of DVT between 20% and 35% using contrast venography and with a rate of symptomatic DVT between 2.3% and 6%. Traumatic cranial injuries have been less well evaluated but the risk is felt to be around 5%. Several specific risk factors have been identified that increase the risk of VTE – paralysis or paresis, a meningioma or malignant tumour, a large tumour, age over 60 years, surgery lasting more than 4 hours, and chemotherapy. Both mechanical methods and LMWHs have shown benefit in reducing VTE in neurosurgery (Grade A) [2]. Both methods decrease the risk by about 50%. Although influencing the uptake of pharmacological thromboprophylaxis, postoperative prophylaxis with a LMWH does not seem to increase the risk of intracranial bleeding (Grade C). However, there is no demonstrated benefit in pre-operative thromboprophylaxis. The customary duration of prophylaxis is 7–10 days, but this has not been scientifically determined.

Prophylaxis against VTE, DVT and PE is a patient safety issue, and options include elastic stockings, IPC stockings, low-dose UFH (5000 IU every 8–12 hours) and LMWH. The risks and benefits associated with different prophylaxis regimens used in the prevention of DVT and PE in neurosurgical procedures have been analysed. Flinn and co-workers [3] found that the incidence of DVT was greater for cranial (7.7%) than spinal procedures (1.5%) and, although IPC devices provided adequate reduction of DVT/PE events in some cranial and combined cranial/spinal series, low-dose subcutaneous UFH or LMWH further reduced the incidence, not always of DVT, but of PE [4,5]. Nevertheless, low-dose heparin-based prophylaxis in cranial and spinal series does carry a risk of minor and major postoperative haemorrhages [3,6–8], including:

- 2–4% in a cranial series;
- 3.4% minor and 3.4% major haemorrhages in a combined cranial/spinal series; and
- a 0.7% incidence of major/minor haemorrhages in a spinal series.

Traumatic closed head injury is an area where evidence is sparse. Norwood et al. [9] concluded that LMWH could be safely administered 24 hours after a head injury complicated by intracranial haemorrhage without an increased risk of haemorrhage progression or new bleeding. Although mechanical prophylaxis has proved effective against DVT and PE in many series, the added efficacy of low-dose heparin regimens has to be weighed against risks of major postoperative haemorrhages and their neurological sequelae [10].

Many neurosurgeons are reluctant to use perioperative anticoagulant prophylaxis, despite its proven success in reducing DVT rates, because of the potentially serious consequences of even a small intracranial bleed. Recent studies have indicated that a combination of GCS and LMWH, started in the postoperative period, significantly reduces the incidence of DVT compared with GCS alone [11]. Postoperative regimens avoid the risk of surgical haemorrhage and appear to offer increased protection for this group of patients.

A survey of 58 consultant neurosurgeons in the UK [12] confirmed that 84.5% regularly used some form of prophylaxis. For all forms of neurosurgery, the most preferred method of prophylaxis was mechanical (GCS or thrombo embolism deterrent stockings [TEDS], and intraoperative pneumatic calf compressors) or, in the postoperative period, a combination of mechanical methods and LMWH. LMWH was rarely administered in the perioperative period. The majority of neurosurgeons believed that TEDS and LMWH reduced postoperative DVT (79% and 90%, respectively) and PE (43% and 67%, respectively), but 29% associated LMWH with bleeding complications. Careful management of anticoagulant thromboprophylaxis provides improved outcomes in the prevention of VTE, but there is still room for improvement, as a minority of neurosurgeons continue to ignore the importance of prophylaxis against thromboembolism in neurosurgery.

Guidelines

The following recommendations were made at the 8th ACCP Conference on Antithrombotic and Thrombolytic Therapy [13]. (A guide to the grading system is provided in Figure 5.2.)

Neurosurgery

- Thromboprophylaxis should be routinely used in patients undergoing major neurosurgery (**Grade 1A**), with optimal use of IPC (**Grade 1A**).
- Acceptable alternatives to the above options are prophylaxis with low-dose UFH (**Grade 2B**) or postoperative LMWH (**Grade 2A**).
- Mechanical prophylaxis (i.e. GCS and/or IPC) and pharmacological prophylaxis (i.e. low-dose UFH or LMWH) should be combined in high-risk neurosurgery patients (**Grade 2B**).

Acute spinal cord injury

- Thromboprophylaxis should be provided for all patients with acute spinal cord injuries (SCIs) (**Grade 1A**).
- In patients with acute SCIs, prophylaxis with LMWH should be commenced once primary haemostasis is evident (**Grade 1B**). The combination of IPC and either low-dose UFH (**Grade 1B**) or LMWH (**Grade 1C**) should be used as alternatives to LMWH.
- IPC and/or GCS should be used when anticoagulant prophylaxis is contraindicated early after injury (**Grade 1A**). Pharmacological thromboprophylaxis should be substituted or added to mechanical thromboprophylaxis when the high risk of bleeding decreases (**Grade 1C**).
- An inferior vena cava filter (IVCF) should NOT be used as primary prophylaxis against PE (**Grade 1C**).
- During the rehabilitation phase following acute SCI, LMWH prophylaxis should be continued or the patient should be converted to an oral vitamin K antagonist (INR target, 2.5; INR range 2.0–3.0) (**Grade 1C**).

NICE recommends that all patients having neurosurgery are offered mechanical prophylaxis and that those with one or more risk factors for VTE should also be offered LMWH or UFH [14]. Pharmacological thromboprophylaxis is contraindicated, however, in patients who have ruptured cranial or spinal malformations, such as brain aneurysms, until the lesion has been secured.

Urological surgery

Because many patients with urological disease are elderly, these patients often have a higher risk than other surgical patients and thromboembolic events are regarded as the most important nonsurgical complication to occur in major urological procedures [15–17]. The incidence of DVT in urological surgery is considered to be broadly similar to that in general surgery, but ranges from 40% in open prostatectomy to 10% in transurethral surgery have been described. However, the available epidemiological data were accumulated approximately 10–30 years ago. Changes in surgical care, earlier postoperative mobilisation of patients and the introduction of various methods of thromboprophylaxis have since resulted in a decrease of the reported rates of thrombosis [18,19]. Published reports in the 1990s range from 1% to 5% of patients undergoing major urological surgery experiencing symptomatic VTE, with fatal PE being occasionally reported [18–22]. The introduction of LMWH as prophylaxis was not shown to be detrimental in either the formation of pelvic lymphoceles or in increased blood loss [23]. There was recognition that certain factors increased the risk of VTE in urology patients. An open procedure had more risk than a transurethral one, whilst other factors (i.e. increased age, general anaesthesia and duration of procedure) were similar to patients undergoing general surgical procedures. There is broad agreement that prophylaxis is required for open procedures and this comes down, at present, to surgeon-specific protocols [24] based upon recognised published guidelines.

Guidelines

The following recommendations were made at the 8th ACCP Conference on Antithrombotic and Thrombolytic Therapy [13].

Urological surgery

- Specific prophylaxis other than early and persistent mobilisation should NOT be used in patients undergoing transurethral or other low-risk urological procedures (**Grade 1A**).
- Routine prophylaxis is recommended for patients undergoing major, open urological procedures (**Grade 1A**). First choice is with low-dose UFH twice daily or three times daily (**Grade 1B**). Acceptable alternatives

include prophylaxis with IPC and/or GCS (**Grade 1B**) or LMWH (**Grade 1C**), fondaparinux (**Grade 1C**), or a combined pharmacological approach with the optimum use of a mechanical method (**Grade 1C**).

- Mechanical prophylaxis with GCS and/or IPC should be used for urological surgery patients who are actively bleeding or are at very high risk for bleeding, at least until the bleeding risk decreases (**Grade 1A**).

- When the bleeding risk decreases, pharmacological thromboprophylaxis should be substituted for or added to mechanical thromboprophylaxis (**Grade 1C**).

The SIGN guidelines include the following recommendations [25]. (A guide to the SIGN grading system is provided in Figure 7.1.)

Major or open urological procedures

- The preferred method of prophylaxis in patients undergoing major or open urological procedures who are at significant risk of VTE (age >40 years or other risk factors) is subcutaneous low-dose UFH (5000 IU, 8–12 hourly) or subcutaneous LMWH (dose as per manufacturer's instructions) (**Grade A**).

- In patients in whom UFH or LMWH are contraindicated, mechanical prophylaxis (GECS ± IPC) can be considered (**Grade B**).

Transurethral resection of the prostate

- In patients undergoing transurethral resection of the prostate who are at increased risk of VTE due to multiple risk factors, antithrombotic prophylaxis with UFH, LMWH or GECS ± IPC should be considered (**Grade C**).

Meanwhile, NICE recommends that mechanical prophylaxis is offered and LMWH is also used in those with one or more risk factors for VTE [14].

Cardiothoracic surgery

Cardiac surgeons recognise the increased risk of VTE following cardiac surgery but again face the quandary of the accepted benefits of LMWH thromboprophylaxis versus a perceived increased risk of bleeding as a result of their use. Several studies have confirmed the high rate of VTE occurring after coronary artery bypass grafting [26–29]. Rates from 3.2% of clinically apparent PE [26] to 17–22% 'clinically silent' DVT [28,29] have been observed, with half the thromboses in the latter study being observed in the leg contralateral to the saphenous vein harvest site. Risk factors for PE included prolonged postoperative recovery, obesity and hyperlipidaemia. It was noted that the adoption of heparin prophylaxis until discharge predicted the absence of DVT after adjustment for immobility.

SIGN grades of evidence	
Level/grade	Clarity and methodological strength of evidence
1++	High-quality meta-analyses, systematic reviews of RCTs, or RCTs with a very low risk of bias
1+	Well-conducted meta-analyses, systematic reviews, or RCTs with a low risk of bias
1−	Meta-analyses, systematic reviews, or RCTs with a high risk of bias
2++	High-quality systematic reviews of case control or cohort studies; or high-quality case control or cohort studies with a very low risk of confounding or bias and a high probability that the relationship is causal
2+	Well-conducted case control or cohort studies with a low risk of confounding or bias and a moderate probability that the relationship is causal
2−	Case control or cohort studies with a high risk of confounding or bias and a significant risk that the relationship is not causal
3	Non-analytic studies; e.g., case reports, case series
4	Expert opinion
A	At least one high-quality meta-analysis, systematic review or RCT rated as 1++, and directly applicable to the target population; or a body of evidence consisting principally of studies rated as 1+, directly applicable to the target population, and demonstrating overall consistency of results
B	A body of evidence including studies rated as 2++, directly applicable to the target population, and demonstrating overall consistency of results; or extrapolated evidence from studies rated as 1++ or 1+
C	A body of evidence including studies rated as 2+, directly applicable to the target population and demonstrating overall consistency of results; or Extrapolated evidence from studies rated as 2++
D	Evidence level 3 or 4; or extrapolated evidence from studies rated as 2+

Figure 7.1 RCT, randomised controlled trials. Reproduced with permission from Scottish Intercollegiate Guidelines Network (SIGN) [25].

Guidelines

The following recommendations have been provided by SIGN [25].

- In patients undergoing major cardiothoracic surgery who are at significant risk of VTE, subcutaneous low-dose UFH or LMWH are recommended. Mechanical prophylaxis (GECS ± IPC) is an alternative (**Grade B**).
- In patients undergoing cardiac surgery, the addition of IPC to heparin prophylaxis should be considered (**Grade A**).
- Aspirin should be discontinued prior to elective cardiac bypass surgery because of the risks of bleeding, and resumed (75–300 mg/day) via nasogastric tube 6 hours following bypass grafting and continued long term in patients with symptomatic arterial disease (**Grade A**).

The following recommendations were made at the 8th ACCP Conference on Antithrombotic and Thrombolytic Therapy [13].

Peripheral vascular surgery
- In patients undergoing vascular surgery who do not have additional thromboembolic risk factors, clinicians should NOT routinely use thromboprophylaxis (**Grade 2B**).
- For patients undergoing major vascular surgical procedures who have additional thromboembolic risk factors, prophylaxis with low-dose UFH, LMWH, or fondaparinux should be used (**Grade 1C**).

The NICE guidelines state that mechanical prophylaxis should be offered and LMWH used in patients with one or more VTE risk factors [14]. It is noted that patients who are already receiving an agent that provides prophylaxis may not need additional pharmacological prophylaxis.

Gynaecological surgery

VTE is an important complication of major gynaecological surgery with rates of DVT, PE and fatal PE similar to those seen after general surgical procedures. Risk factors for the development of VTE in relation to gynaecological surgery include malignancy, age, previous VTE, prior pelvic radiotherapy and the use of an abdominal surgical approach. Furthermore, in women with gynaecological malignancies, venous compression by the tumour or venous intimal damage secondary to surgery or radiotherapy also increase the risk of VTE. Finally, surgery in such individuals is often lengthy with a slow postoperative recovery.

The ACCP guidelines [13] make the following recommendations.

Gynaecology
- In low-risk patients undergoing minor gynaecological surgery, no specific measures are recommended other than early and persistent mobilisation (**Grade 1A**).
- In patients undergoing laparoscopic gynaecological surgery in whom additional risk factors for VTE are present, thromboprophylaxis with either low-dose UFH, LMWH, IPC or GCS should be used (**Grade 1C**).
- In patients undergoing major gynaecological surgery but no other risk factors, the recommendations include low-dose UFH (**Grade 1A**), LMWH (**Grade 1A**) or IPC started immediately before surgery and used continuously whilst the patient is not ambulant (**Grade 1B**).

- In patients undergoing major gynaecological surgery for malignancy or with additional VTE risk factors, low-dose UFH three times daily or LMWH should be used (**Grade 1A**). Alternative considerations include IPC started before surgery and continued until discharge (**Grade 1A**) or a combination of low-dose UFH or LMWH with IPS or GCS (**Grade 1C**). For patients at very high risk (age >60, undergoing cancer surgery or a previous VTE), thromboprophylaxis with LMWH for up to 28 days after hospital discharge should be considered (**Grade 2C**).

In practice, most women undergoing gynaecological surgery will receive once-daily LMWH (e.g. enoxaparin 40 mg once daily or dalteparin 5000 IU once daily), GCS and early mobilisation. NICE recommends mechanical prophylaxis in all women undergoing gynaecological procedures, with added LMWH if they have one or more risk factors for VTE [14].

Patients with mechanical heart valves

The management of patients with mechanical heart valves who require surgery is a common clinical problem.

Risk stratification for patients with mechanical heart valves

Patients with mechanical heart valves are at increased risk of valvular and intra-cardiac thrombus formation in addition to arterial thromboembolism including stroke and systemic embolism.

Most estimates of arterial thromboembolic risk are derived from studies in which patients were receiving either no antithrombotic therapy or treatment that is currently considered suboptimal. There are little data available on the risk of thromboembolism in patients who have modern prostheses and have not received antithrombotic therapy over an extended time period. In the absence of such data it is sensible to err on the side of caution when recommending anticoagulant treatment or thromboprophylaxis for such patients.

High-risk patients (>10%/annum) include:
- Mitral valve prosthesis
- Older-generation (caged-ball or tilting disk) aortic valve prosthesis
- A recent (< 6 months) stroke or transient ischaemic attack.

Moderate-risk patients (4–10%/annum) include:
- Bileaflet aortic valve prosthesis and one of the following:

- Atrial fibrillation
- Prior stroke or transient ischaemic attack
- Other risk factors for stroke (hypertension, diabetes, congestive heart failure, age >75 years).

Low-risk patients (<4%/annum) are essentially those that do not fall into either of the above groups and include those with a bileaflet aortic valve prosthesis without atrial fibrillation and no other risk factors for stroke.

In individuals with a bioprosthetic valve, the risk of systemic arterial thromboembolism is increased in patients with:

- Atrial fibrillation
- Previous systemic embolism
- Evidence of left atrial thrombus at surgery
- A mitral valve prosthesis (for three months following surgery)

Management:

High-risk patients:

In patients who are perceived at being of high risk of thrombosis bridging therapy is recommended. Subcutaneous therapeutic LMWH is generally preferable to intravenous UFH.

Moderate-risk patients:

In patients with a mechanical heart valve at moderate risk for VTE, bridging therapy with either therapeutic-dose subcutaneous LMWH, therapeutic-dose intravenous UFH, or low-dose subcutaneous LMWH is preferable to no treatment.

Low-risk patients:

In patients with a mechanical heart valve thought to be at low risk for VTE, bridging therapy with low-dose subcutaneous LMWH is preferable to no treatment.

References

1. Kamphuisen PW, Agnelli G, Sebastianelli M. Prevention of venous thromboembolism after acute ischemic stroke. J Thromb Haemost 2005; 3:1187–1194.
2. Payen JF, Faillot T, Audibert G, et al. Thromboprophylaxis in neurosurgery and head trauma. Ann Fr Anesth Reanim 2005; 24:921–927.
3. Flinn WR, Sandager GP, Silva MB Jr, et al. Prospective surveillance for perioperative venous thrombosis. Experience in 2643 patients. Arch Surg 1996; 131:472–480.
4. Stephens PH, Healy MT, Smith M, et al. Prophylaxis against thromboembolism in neurosurgical patients: a survery of current practice in the United Kingdom. Br J Neurosurg 1995; 9:159–163.
5. Streiff, MB. Vena caval filters: a review for intensive care speciailists. J Intensive Care Med 2003; 18:59–79.
6. Auguste KI, Quinones-Hinojosa A, Gadkary C, et al. Incidence of venous thromboembolism in patients undergoing craniotomy and motor mapping for glioma without intraoperative mechanical prophylaxis to the controlateral leg. J Neurosurg 2003; 99:680–684.
7. Black PM, Baker MF, Snook CP. Experience with external pneumatic calf compression in neurology and neurosurgery. Neurosurgery 1986; 18:440–445.
8. Brambilla S, Ruosi C, La Maida GA, et al. Prevention of venous thromboembolism in spinal surgery. Eur Spine J 2004; 13:1–8.
9. Norwood SH, McAuley CE, Berne JD, et al. Prospective evalution of the safety of enoxaparin prophylaxis for venous thromboembolism in patients with intracranial haemorrhagic injuries. Arch Surg2002. 137:696–702.
10. Epstein NE. A review of the risks and benefits of differing prophylaxis regimens for the treatment of deep venous thrombosis and pulmonary embolism in neurosurgery. Surg Neurol 2005; 64:295–301.
11. Nurmohamed MT. Thromboprophylaxis in neurosurgical patients. Semin Hematol 2000; 37(Suppl 5):15–18.
12. Gnanalingham KK, Holland JP. Attitudes to the use of prophylaxis for thromboembolism in neurosurgical patients. J Clin Neurosci 2003; 10:467–469.
13. Geerts WH, Bergqvist D, Pineo GF, et al. Prevention of venous thromboembolism. American College of Chest Physicians Evidence-Based Clinical Practice Guidelines. Chest 2008; 133(6, Suppl):381S–453S.
14. National Institute of Clinical Excellence. Venous thromboembolism - reducing the risk NICE clinical guidelines CG92 (January 2010). Available at: www.nice.org.uk/nicemedia/pdf/CG92NICEGuidance.pdf.
15. Brenner DW, Fogle MA, Schellhammer PF. VTE. J Urol 1989; 142:1403–1411.
16. Kibel AS, Loughlin KR. Pathogenesis and prophylaxis of postoperative thromboembolic disease in urological pelvic surgery. J Urol 1995; 153:1763–1774.
17. Koch MO, Smith JA. Low molecular weight heparin and radical prostatectomy: a prospective analysis of safety and side effects. Prostate Cancer Prostatic Dis1997 1:101–104.
18. Dillioglugil O, Leibman BD, Leibman NS, et al. Risk factors for complications and morbidity after radical retropubic prostatectomy. J Urol 1997; 157:1760–1767.
19. Heinzer H, Hammerer P, Graefen M, et al. Thromboembolic complication rate after radical retropubic prostatectomy: impact of routine ultrasonography for the detection of pelvic lymphocoeles and hematomas. Eur Urol 1998; 33:86–90.
20. Rossignol G, Leandri P, Gautier JR, et al. Radical retropubic prostatectomy: complications and quality of life (429 cases, 1983–1989). Eur Urol 1991; 19:186–191.
21. Cisek LJ, Walsh PC. Thromboembolic complications following radical retropubic prostatectomy: influence of external sequential pneumatic compression devices. Urology 1993; 42:406–408.

22. Leibovitch I, Foster RS, Wass JL, et al. Color Dopper flow imaging for deep venous thrombosis screening in patients undergoing pelvic lymphadenectomy and radical retropubic prostatectomy for prostatic carcinoma. J Urol 1995; 153:1866–1869.

23. Sieber PR, Rommel FM, Agusta VE, et al. Is heparin contraindicated in pelvic lymphadenectomy and radical prostatectomy? J Urol1997 158:869–871.

24. Koya MP, Manoharan M, Kim SS, et al. Venous thromboembolism in radical prostatectomy: is heparinoid prophylaxis warranted? BJU Intl 2005; 96:1019–1021.

25. Scottish and Collegiate Guideline Network (SIGN). Prophylaxis of Venous Thromboembolism. London, SIGN publication, 2002; no. 62. Available at: www.sign.ac.uk/guidelines.

26. Josa M, Siouffi SY, Silverman AB, et al. Pulmonary embolism after cardiac surgery. J Am Coll Cardiol 1993; 21:990–996.

27. Shammas NW. Pulmonary embolus after coronary artery bypass surgery: a review of the literature. Clin Cardiol 2000; 23:637–644.

28. Goldhaber SZ, Hirsch DR, MacDougall RC, et al. Prevention of venous thrombosis after coronary artery bypass surgery (a randomised trial comparing two mechanical prophylaxis strategies). Am J Cardiol 1995; 76:993–996.

29. Ambrosetti M, Salerno M, Zambelli M, et al. Deep vein thrombosis among patients entering cardiac rehabilitation after coronary artery bypass surgery – clinical investigations. Chest 2004; 125:191–196.

Chapter 8

Thromboprophylaxis in patients on oral anticoagulant therapy

The perioperative management of patients on oral anticoagulants is a common clinical problem. Many patients can undergo dental surgery (including extractions), joint and soft tissue aspirations/injections, cataract surgery and diagnostic endoscopies without any alteration to their anticoagulant regimen. For other invasive and surgical procedures, oral anticoagulation needs to be withheld and a decision made regarding whether to introduce bridging therapy with either intravenous UFH or subcutaneous LMWH.

The following recommendations are based upon the ACCP and the British Committee for Standards in Haematology (BCSH) guidelines.

1. **Stopping oral anticoagulants prior to invasive and/or surgical procedures:** Oral anticoagulants should be discontinued 5 days prior to surgery to allow normalisation of the INR. Oral anticoagulants can be re-started 12–24 hours after surgery i.e. the evening of surgery or the following morning assuming there is adequate haemostasis.

2. **High-risk patients:** In patients who are perceived as being at high risk of thrombosis, which includes patients with a mechanical heart valve, atrial fibrillation or recurrent or recent VTE, bridging therapy is recommended. Subcutaneous therapeutic LMWH is generally preferable to intravenous UFH.

3. **Moderate-risk patients:** In patients with a mechanical heart valve, atrial fibrillation or recurrent VTE at moderate risk for VTE, bridging therapy with either therapeutic-dose subcutaneous LMWH, therapeutic-dose intravenous UFH, or low-dose subcutaneous LMWH is preferable to no treatment.

4. Low-risk patients: In patients with a mechanical heart valve, atrial fibrillation or recurrent VTE and thought to be at low risk for VTE, bridging therapy with low-dose subcutaneous LMWH is preferable to no treatment.

The stratification of patients into those who are at high, moderate and low risk for thromboembolic disease is difficult. The ACCP guidelines [1] and others have used available data to provide guidelines on thrombotic risk associated with various disorders. For a table defining three risk catagories for thromboemoblism see Figure 8.1.

5. Stopping heparin prior to any invasive and/or surgical procedure: In patients receiving bridging anticoagulation with subcutaneous therapeutic LMWH, the last dose of a LMWH should be given 24 hours prior to any invasive and/or surgical procedure and with a 50% reduction, i.e. half the daily dose. In patients who are on intravenous UFH, the infusion should be stopped 4 hours prior to any invasive and/or surgical procedure. Standard low-dose thromboprophylaxis with a LMWH, (e.g. enoxaparin 40 mg subcutaneous once daily) can be given to patients to cover surgery when therapeutic anticoagulants have been discontinued.

6. Re-starting heparin following an invasive and/or surgical procedure: In patients undergoing a minor surgical or invasive procedure and in whom heparin has been stopped prior to surgery, assuming adequate haemostasis, therapeutic subcutaneous LMWH can be reinstituted approximately 24 hours after surgery. In practice this is usually the day following the procedure.

For patients undergoing more major surgery or in whom there is a high risk of bleeding associated with the procedure, then the re-introduction of heparin should be delayed for 48–72 hours or when adequate haemostasis has been achieved. For a table summarising who should receive bridging therapy see Figure 8.2.

In patients on bridging therapy there is little if any role for measuring anti-Xa assays.

Which patients on warfarin should receive heparin bridging before surgery?

High risk for thromboembolism: bridging advised

Known hypercoagulable state as documented by a thromboembolic event and one of the following:

- Protein C deficiency

- Protein S deficiency

- Antithrombin deficiency

- Homozygous factor V Leiden mutation

- Antiphospholipid-antibody syndrome

- Hypercoagulable state suggested by recurrent (two or more) arterial or idiopathic venous thromboembolic events (not including primary atherosclerotic events, such as stroke or myocardial infarction due to intrinsic cerebrovascular or coronary disease)

- Venous or arterial thromboembolism within the preceding 1–3 months

- Rheumatic atrial fibrillation

- Acute intracardiac thrombus visualized by echocardiogram

- Atrial fibrillation plus mechanical heart valve in any position

- Older mechanical valve model (single-disc or ball-in-cage) in mitral position

- Recently placed mechanical valve (<3 months)

- Atrial fibrillation with history of cardioembolism

Intermediate risk for thromboembolism: bridging on a case-by-case basis

Cerebrovascular disease with multiple (two or more) strokes or transient ischaemic attacks without risk factors for cardiac embolism

Newer mechanical valve model (e.g. St. Jude) in mitral position

Older mechanical valve model in aortic position

Atrial fibrillation without a history of cardiac embolism but with multiple risks for cardiac embolism (e.g. ejection fraction < 40%, diabetes, hypertension, nonrheumatic valvular heart disease, transmural myocardial infarction within preceding month)

Venous thromboembolism >3–6 months ago*

Low risk for thromboembolism: bridging not advised

One remote venous thromboembolism (>6 months ago)*

Intrinsic cerebrovascular disease (such as carotid atherosclerosis) without recurrent strokes or transient ischemic attacks

Atrial fibrillation without multiple risks for cardiac embolism

Newer-model prosthetic valve in aortic position

Figure 8.1 Reproduced with permission from Jaffer et al [3]. *For patients with a history of venous thromboembolism undergoing major surgery, consideration can be given to postoperative bridging therapy only (without preoperative bridging).

Cleveland Clinic Anticoagulation Clinic protocol for LMWH as a bridge to surgery in patients on warfarin

Inclusion criteria

Age >18 years, needing to undergo therapy with LMWH

Treating physician thinks patient needs bridging therapy

Medically and haemodynamically stable

Scheduled for elective procedure or surgery

Exclusion criteria

Allergy to UFH or LMWH

Weight >150 kg

Pregnant woman with a mechanical valve

History of bleeding disorder or intracranial haemorrhage

Creatinine clearance <30 mL/minute

Gastrointestinal bleeding within the last 10 days

Major trauma or stroke within the past 2 weeks

History of heparin-induced thrombocytopenia or severe thrombocytopenia

Language barrier

Potential for medication noncompliance

Unsuitable home environment to support therapy

Severe liver disease

Before surgery

If preoperative international normalized ratio (INR) is 2.0–3.0, stop warfarin 5 days before surgery (i.e. hold four doses)

If preoperative INR is 3.0–4.5, stop warfarin 6 days before surgery (hold five doses)

Start LMWH 36 hours after last warfarin dose, ie:

- Enoxaparin 1 mg/kg subcutaneously every 12 hours,* or
- Enoxaparin 1.5 mg/kg subcutaneously every 24 hours, or
- Dalteparin 120 U/kg subcutaneously every 12 hours, or
- Dalteparin 200 U/kg subcutaneously every 24 hours, or
- Tinzaparin 175 U/kg subcutaneously every 24 hours

Give last dose of LMWH approximately 24 hours before procedure

Educate patient in self-injection and provide with written instructions

Discuss plan with surgeon and anaesthesiologist

Check INR in morning of surgery to ensure that it is <1.5, or in some cases (e.g. neurological surgery) <1.2

Figure 8.2 Reproduced with permission from Jaffer et al [3]. *For patients with a history of venous thromboembolism undergoing major surgery, consideration can be given to postoperative bridging therapy only (without preoperative bridging).

After surgery

Restart LMWH approximately 24 hours after procedure or consider thromboprophylactic dose of LMWH on first postoperative day if patient is at high risk for bleeding

Discuss above with surgeon

Start warfarin at patient's preoperative dose on postoperative day 1

Daily prothrombin time and INR until patient is discharged and periodically thereafter until

INR is in the therapeutic range

Daily phone follow-up with patient by the pharmacist to assess for adverse effects such as bleeding

Complete blood cell count with platelets on day 3 and day 7

Discontinue LMWH when INR is 2–3 for 2 consecutive days

Figure 8.2 *Continued*.

References

1. Douketis JD, Berger PB, Dunn AS, et al. The peri-operative management of antithrombotic therapy. Chest 2008;133:299–339.
2. Baglin TP, Keeling DN, Watson HG. Guidelines on oral anticoagulation: third edition. Brit J Haem 1998;101(2):374–87 and 2006;132(3): 277–85
3. Jaffer AK, Brotman DJ, Chuk Wumerije N. When patients on warfarin need surgery. Clev Clin J Med 2003;70:973–984.

Chapter 9

The pharmacoeconomics of surgical thromboprophylaxis

As mentioned earlier, patients undergoing surgical procedures, particularly operations such as hip or knee arthroplasty, face an increased risk of thrombotic events, including DVT, PE and major bleeding. There are a range of interventions designed to prevent such complications, ranging from compression stockings through to warfarin and LMWH. While the clinical efficacy of these prophylactic interventions has been widely explored, one of the main issues facing physicians is how to balance the clinical needs of patients with the costs of such therapies in healthcare systems. Several key trials on the cost effectiveness of thromboprophylaxis undergoing elective surgery have been conducted. These trials focus on the treatment of patients in a range of settings in Western Europe and the USA. Although the findings are therefore not directly comparable, they reveal that, despite treatment with LMWHs resulting in higher direct healthcare costs, the subsequent reductions in thromboembolic complications are substantial. This typically leads to low costs per life - or quality-adjusted life-years saved, as well as overall healthcare savings.

Enoxaparin versus warfarin

Garcia-Zozaya [1] carried out an economic analysis of longer-term thromboprophylaxis in patients undergoing total hip and knee arthroplasty in the USA. Thromboprophylaxis, which was either warfarin 10 mg followed by 5 mg daily or enoxaparin 30 mg twice daily, was started within 12 hours of surgery and then continued for 15 days. The total cumulative costs per patient with warfarin were US$971.77 compared with US$925.38 when using LMWH. This gave an overall cost saving per patient with enoxaparin of US$46.39.

Enoxaparin versus unfractionated heparin

Drummond et al. [2] performed an analysis combining clinical effectiveness and cost data on a hypothetical population of UK patients undergoing elective hip surgery. The model was based on either enoxaparin 40 mg once daily given 12 hours before surgery or UFH 5000 IU every 8 hours initiated 2 hours before surgery, with treatment continued until discharge.

The analysis revealed that the expected mortality per 1000 patients would be 9.07 with UFH versus 4.54 for enoxaparin, giving a difference of 4.53. With a cost per 1000 patients treated of £1,223,839 (US$ 250,666) for UFH compared with £103,543 (US$190,358) for enoxaparin, the cost saving with enoxaparin was calculated at £20,296 (US$37,313) per 1000 patients treated.

Hawkins et al. [3] looked at the results of three published US trials on thromboprophylaxis to compare prophylaxis for 7 days with either enoxaparin 60 mg/day or UFH 15,000 IU/day in patients undergoing total hip replacement surgery. The three trials revealed that enoxaparin resulted in fewer DVT events per 1000 patients in comparison with UFH, with reductions of 22, 30 and 89 events. The cost analysis showed that the cost per additional event avoided with enoxaparin in the three trials was US$2273, US$1176 and US$494 respectively.

Marchetti et al. [4] examined a meta-analysis of trials published in Europe between 1982 and 1988 to create a model of a typical 67-year-old patient undergoing elective hip replacement to compare a 2- or 4-week prophylaxis regimen containing either enoxaparin 40 mg once daily or UFH 5000 IU three-times daily. The quality-adjusted life expectancy with enoxaparin was 13.40 versus 13.33 for UFH, which resulted in an estimated two lives saved for every 1000 patients treated with enoxaparin. Given overall costs for enoxaparin therapy of US$2208, compared with US$2283 for UFH, the average cost saving per patient with enoxaparin therapy was US$75.

Enoxaparin versus ardeparin

Wade et al. [5] undertook a cost analysis of trials conducted between 1994 and 1996 involving patients undergoing knee arthroplasty in the USA and involving ardeparin 50 IU/kg twice daily versus enoxaparin 30 mg twice daily or enoxaparin 40 mg administered once daily. The incidences of DVT, proximal DVT, PE and major bleeding among patients treated with ardeparin were 28.0%, 2.0%, 1.0% and 5.2%, respectively. This compared with respective rates for enoxaparin of 29.5%, 5.8%, 0.2% and 2.2%. The overall costs per 1000 patients with ardeparin were US$613,647, versus US$709,923 for enoxaparin 30 mg twice daily and US$323,429 for enoxaparin 40 mg. This gave an overall cost saving for enoxaparin 40 mg of US$290 in comparison with ardeparin and US$386 versus enoxaparin 30 mg twice daily.

Continued enoxaparin therapy

Detournay et al. [6] performed a cost data analysis of a hypothetical population of patients in France undergoing total hip replacement who were treated with enoxaparin 40 mg, and then given either enoxaparin or placebo for 3 weeks. Continued enoxaparin therapy resulted in significant reductions in outcome measures versus placebo, with 16,012–21,222 thromboembolic events avoided preventing a median of 601–783 deaths. More importantly, there was an incremental cost effectiveness for every death avoided with enoxaparin of between US$23,247 and US$36,031.

Berqvist and Jönsson [7] carried out a cost-effectiveness analysis of an earlier thromboprophylaxis study of Swedish patients undergoing elective hip replacement. The participants were treated with enoxaparin for an average of 9 days, and then randomised to enoxaparin 40 mg once daily or placebo for between 19 and 23 days following discharge. The event rate of DVT with placebo was more than twice that seen with enoxaparin, at 0.3435 versus 0.1603, respectively, while the overall rate of clinical events was 0.0687 versus 0.0153. With combined costs per patient of SEK319,500 (US$43,283) for the enoxaparin group and SEK844,500 (US$114,405) for placebo, the net saving per patient with continued enoxaparin therapy was calculated to be SEK3400 (US$460).

Davies et al. [8] focused on patients in the UK, conducting a cost-effectiveness analysis of patients undergoing elective hip surgery, who were treated with enoxaparin during the index hospital admission only (standard therapy) or given the drug during the index hospital admission and for 21 days post discharge (extended therapy). Extended therapy resulted in a survival per 1000 patients of 999, compared with 993 for standard therapy, along with 10,066 life-years gained versus 10,009 for standard therapy, and 7476 quality-adjusted life-years (QALY) versus 7434 for standard therapy. Further analysis showed that the cost per life gained with enoxaparin was £42,898 (US$78,887), with £4257 (US$7824) per life-year gained and £5732 (US$10,537) per QALY gained.

Dabigatran versus enoxaparin

Wolowacz et al. [9] compared the cost-effectiveness of oral dabigatran 220 mg once daily and enoxaparin 40 mg once daily in patients undergoing total knee or total knee replacement surgery, at a duration of prophylaxis of 6–10 days and 28–35 days, respectively. A decision tree was used to model the 10-week acute postsurgical phase, while long-term events were modeled using a Markov process. This revealed that, although bleeding rates did not differ significantly between dabigatran- and enoxaparin-treated patients, costs were reduced with dabigatran in both total hip and total knee replacement surgery, largely due to differences in administration costs. The combined costs of prophylaxis, including drugs and administration was £137 for dabigatran versus £237 for enoxaparin for total hip replacement patients, while the costs in total knee replacement patients were £30 and £38, respectively. Furthermore, at a willingness-to-pay threshold of £20,000 per QALY, the probability for the cost-effectiveness of dabigatran was 75% in total knee replacement and 97% in total hip replacement [9].

Conclusion

The above results show that, in patients undergoing elective surgery, treatment with LMWHs leads to cost benefits in comparison with other forms of thromboprophylaxis. Enoxaparin therapy, in particular, leads to cost savings when compared with not only warfarin, but also UFH and ardeparin. Furthermore, continuing enoxaparin therapy beyond the index hospital admission in elective surgery patients improves both the outcomes and the costs incurred, resulting in substantial savings.

However, it appears that dabigatran provides cost savings compared with enoxaparin, while a achieving a comparable safety profile.

References

1. Garcia-Zozaya I. Warfarin vs enoxaparin for deep venous thrombosis prophylaxis after total hip and total knee arthroplasty: a US cost comparison. J KY Med Assoc 1998; 96:143–148.
2. Drummond M, Aristides M, Davies L, et al. United Kingdom economic evaluation of standard heparin and enoxaparin for prophylaxis against deep vein thrombosis in elective hip surgery. Br J Surg 1994; 81:1742–1746.
3. Hawkins DW, Langley PC, Krueger KP, et al. Pharmacoeconomic model of enoxaparin versus heparin for prevention of deep vein thrombosis after total hip replacement in a US managed care setting. Am J Health-Syst Pharm 1997; 54:1185–1190.
4. Marchetti M, Liberato NL, Ruperto N, et al. Long-term cost-effectiveness of enoxaparin versus unfractionated heparin for the prophylaxis of venous thromboembolism in elective hip replacement in Europe. Haematologica 1999; 84:730–737.
5. Wade WE. Cost analysis of ardeparin versus enoxaparin for the prophylaxis of deep vein thrombosis after knee arthroplasty in the US. Clin Ther 1998; 20:347–351.
6. Detournay B, Planes A, Vochelle N, et al. Cost effectiveness of enoxaparin in prolonged prophylaxis against deep vein thrombosis after total hip replacement in France. Pharmacoeconomics 1988; 13:81–89.
7. Bergqvist D, Jönsson B. Cost-effectiveness of prolonged administration of enoxaparin for the prevention of deep venous thrombosis following total hip replacement in Sweden. Value Health 1999; 2:288–294.
8. Davies LM, Richardson GA, Cohen AT. UK Economic evaluation of enoxaparin as postdischarge prophylaxis for deep vein thrombosis (DVT) in elective hip surgery. Value Health 2000; 3:397–406.
9. Wolowacz SE, Roskell NS, Maciver F. Economic evaluation of dabigatran etexilate for the prevention of venous thromboembolism after total knee and hip replacement surgery. Clin Ther 2009; 31:194–212.

Chapter 10

Thromboprophylaxis in pregnancy

Introduction

Pregnancy is associated with a tenfold increased risk of VTE compared to the nonpregnant woman and this risk may be higher in some women because of the presence of additional risk factors (Figure 10.1) [1]. Thromboembolic disease remains the leading cause of maternal death in the UK [2]. This risk is significantly increased after caesarean section and national guidelines in the UK have been published in an attempt to reduce morbidity and mortality [1].

As the absolute risk of VTE in pregnancy is low, it is recommended that all women should undergo an assessment of risk factors for VTE either before pregnancy or in early pregnancy to establish which women would benefit from pharmacological thromboprophylaxis. This assessment should be repeated if the woman is admitted to hospital or develops other related problems. The risk of thrombosis exists from the beginning of the first trimester, whereas the antenatal booking visit is often scheduled at the end of the first trimester.

Women at high risk of VTE, including those with previous confirmed VTE or who are on long-term anticoagulants for recurrent VTE or who have metal heart valves require pre-pregnancy counselling with a prospective management plan.

Guidelines for thromboprophylaxis during pregnancy

RCOG guidelines for thromboprophylaxis during pregnancy and the puerperium

The RCOG guidelines stratify women on the basis of individual risk factors and the recommendations for thromboprophylaxis are based upon these (Figure 10.2). However, regardless of their risk of VTE, immobilisation of women during pregnancy, labour and the puerperium should be minimised and dehydration should be avoided.

Risk factors for VTE in pregnancy and the puerperium*

Pre-existing	New onset or transient
Previous VTE	Surgical procedure in pregnancy or puerperium (e.g. evacuation of retained products of conception, postpartum sterilisation)
Thrombophilia	Hyperemesis
1. Congenital	Dehydration
Antithrombin deficiency	Ovarian hyperstimulation syndrome
Protein C deficiency	Severe infection (e.g. pyelonephritis)
Protein S deficiency	Immobility (>4 days bed rest)
Factor V Leiden	Pre-eclampsia
Prothrombin G20210A gene variant	Long-haul travel
2. Acquired (antiphospholipid syndrome)	Prolonged hospital admission
Lupus anticoagulant	Excessive blood loss at delivery (PPH >1 L or requiring a blood transfusion)
Anticardiolipin antibodies	Prolonged labour‡
Anti-β2 GPI antibodies	Midcavity instrumental delivery‡
Age ≥35 years	Immobility after delivery‡
Obesity (BMI >30 kg/m²) either pre-pregnancy or in early pregnancy	
Parity >4	
Gross varicose veins	
Paraplegia	
Sickle cell disease	
Intravenous drug use	
Inflammatory disorders (e.g. inflammatory bowel disease)	
Some medical disorders (e.g. nephrotic syndrome, significant proteinuria, certain cardiac diseases)	
Myeloproliferative disorders (e.g. essential thrombocytothaemia, polycythaemia vera)	

Figure 10.1 *Although these are all accepted as thromboembolic risk factors, there are few data to support the degree of increased risk associated with many of them. † These risk factors are potentially reversible and may develop at later stages in gestation than the initial risk assessment or may resolve; an ongoing individual risk assessment is important. ‡Risk factors specific to postpartum venous thromboembolism (VTE) only. BMI, body mass index. Adapted from Royal College of Obstetricians and Gynaecologists guidelines [1].

VTE during pregnancy has an equal distribution throughout gestation and if a decision is made to initiate thromboprophylaxis antenatally (Figure 10.3), this should begin as early in pregnancy as practical.

Once antenatal treatment is initiated it should continue until delivery unless a specific risk factor is removed or disappears. Postpartum thromboprophylaxis should be given as soon as possible after delivery, provided that there is no postpartum haemorrhage.

The prothrombotic changes in pregnancy are maximal immediately following delivery and treatment with LMWH should, therefore, continue during labour. For women who are on therapeutic doses of LMWH, this should be reduced to a prophylactic dose 24–48 hours prior to delivery. This may necessitate a planned delivery and careful coordination with the obstetricians and obstetric anaesthestis is essential. LMWH should be omitted on the day of a planned caesarean section or induction of labour.

Epidural anaesthesia should not be used until at least 12 hours after the last prophylactic dose of LMWH. When a woman presents whilst on a therapeutic regimen of LMWH, regional techniques should not be employed for at least 24 hours following the last dose of LMWH. LMWH should not be given for at least 4 hours after the epidural catheter has been inserted or removed (or 6 hours if either insertion or removal were traumatic), and the cannula should not be removed within 10–12 hours of the most recent injection.

The most recent guidance issued by the RCOG notes that any woman suspected of having VTE should undergo objective testing and treatment with LMWH, unless this is strongly contraindicated or proven unnecessary [4]. The RCOG also states that the evidence suggests that LMWH is a 'safe alternative' to UFH during pregnancy and that it does not cross the placenta. Treatment should be continued throughout pregnancy and continue for at least 6 weeks postnatally or until the patient has been given therapy for a minimum of 3 months.

The RCOG guidelines are sumarised in Figures 10.4 and 10.5.

ACCP guidelines for the prevention of VTE in pregnancy

The ACCP guidelines are similar to those of the RCOG and are summarised in Figure 10.6 [5].

Pharmacological thromboprophylaxis in pregnancy: agents

Unfractionated heparin

Whilst UFH has been shown to be effective as a thromboprophylactic agent, it is associated with more side effects (heparin-induced thrombocytopenia and osteoporosis) and possibly more bleeding complications than the LMWHs and is, therefore, less commonly used than the LMWHs. However, UFH has a shorter half-life than LMWH and there is more complete reversal with protamine sulphate.

Thromboprophylaxis during pregnancy and the puerperium

Risk group	Thromboprophylaxis
Women with a previous single VTE (Unprovoked, thrombophilia, family history of VTE or oestrogen related VTE)	These women should be considered to be at high risk of VTE in pregnancy and should be offered antenatal and postpartum throboprophylaxis with a LMWH
	In women with a temporary risk factor that has now resolved, it may be reasonable to omit antenatal thromboprophylaxis but consider postpartum thromboprophylaxis with a LMWH
Women with inherited thrombophilia but no previous VTE	Women should be stratified according to the level of risk associated with their thrombophilic defect. Women with deficiencies of antithrombin, homozygous defects or combined defects should be considered at high risk of VTE and should be offered antenatal and postpartum thromboprophylaxis with a LMWH
	Women with a 'low-risk' thrombophilia defect (e.g. heterozygosity for the factor V Leiden mutations, the prothrombin G20210A mutation) and no other risk factors for VTE in pregnancy should be monitored. Thromboprophylaxis may be indicated if their risks change during pregnancy
Women with APS	Pregnant women with APS and previous thromboses should receive antenatal and postnatal thromboprophylaxis with a LMWH
	Women on long-term anticoagulation with warfarin due to APS must be changed to therapeutic anticoagulation with a LMWH as soon as a pregnancy test is positive. These women require careful pre-pregnancy counselling
Women with no history of VTE or thrombophilia	Women with 3 or more persisting risk factors (figure 9.1) should be considered for thromboprophylaxis with a LMWH antenatally and for 7 days postpartum
	Women with fewer than 3 risk factors may not require formal thromboprophylaxis. Obesity is a strong risk factor for VTE in pregnancy and the risk of VTE in these women must be assessed
Women who have a ceasarian section	At least 7 days postpartum thromboprophylaxis with a LMWH. In women with persisting risk factors, including an elevated BMI, thromboprophylaxis can be extended for up to 6 weeks

Figure 10.2 APS, antiphospholipid syndrome; BMI, body mass index; LMWH, low-molecular-weight heparin; VTE, venous thromboembolism.

Antenatal prophylactic and therapeutic doses of LMWH			
Prophylaxis	**Enoxaparin**	**Dalteparin**	**Tinzaparin***
Normal body weight (50–90 kg)	40 mg daily	5000 units daily	4500 units daily
Body weight <50 kg	20 mg daily	2500 units daily	3500 units daily
Body weight >90 kg†	40 mg 12-hourly	5000 units 12-hourly	4500 units 12-hourly
Higher prophylactic dose	40 mg 12-hourly	5000 units 12-hourly	4500 units 12-hourly
Therapeutic dose	1 mg/kg 12-hourly	90 units/kg 12-hourly	90 units/kg 12-hourly

Figure 10.3 *The dosage schedules for tinzaparin differ from the manufacturer's recommendation of once-daily dosage. †Body mass index >30 in early pregnancy. Dosages taken from RCOG [1].

Low-molecular-weight heparins

LMWHs are the agents of choice for antenatal thromboprophylaxis. They are effective and safer than UFH in pregnancy. In general, monitoring of anti-Xa levels is not indicated when LMWHs are used for thromboprophylaxis. However, in antithrombin deficiency, higher doses of LMWH and monitoring of anti-Xa levels may be necessary.

Heparin-induced thrombocytopenia is rare with the LMWHs but, in women receiving therapeutic anticoagulation with a LMWH monitoring of the platelet count is recommended every 2 days for the initial 14 days of treatment. In other patients monitoring of the platelet count 1 week after starting treatment is recommended.

Allergic skin reactions to UFH and LMWH are rare but can occur. Switching to a different LMWH preparation or to a heparinoid (danaparoid) may be necessary.

Aspirin

Low-dose aspirin appears safe in pregnancy, although its use as a thromboprophylactic agent is questionable. Aspirin is often combined with a LMWH in women with antiphospholipid syndrome and recurrent miscarriage.

Dextran

Dextran should be avoided in pregnancy. It can cause anaphylaxis, which can kill the fetus.

Antenatal assessment and management
(to be assessed at booking and repeated if admitted)

Single previous VTE + • Thrombophilia or family history • Unprovoked/estrogen-related previous recurrent VTE (> 1)	**High risk** Requires antenatal prophylaxis with LMWH Refer to trust-nominated thrombosis in pregnancy expert/team
Single previous VTE with no family history or thrombophilia Thrombophilia + no VTE Medical co morbidities, e.g. heart or lung disease, SLE, cancer, imflammatory conditions, nephritic syndrome, sickle cell disease, intravenous drug user Surgical procedure, e.g. appendicectomy	**Intermediate risk** Consider antenatal prophylaxis with LMWH Seek trust-nominated thrombosis in pregnancy expert/team advice Obstetric thromboprophylaxis risk assessment and management
Age > 35 years Obesity (BMI > 30kg/m2) Parity ≥ 3 Smoker Gross varicose veins Current systemic infection Immobility, e.g. paraplegia, SPD, long-distance travel Pre-eclampsia Dehydration/hyperemesis/OHSS Multiple pregnancy or ART	3 or more risk factors 2 or more if admitted < 3 risk factors **Lower risk** Mobilisation and avoidance of dehydration

Antenatal and postnatal prophylactic dose of LMWH
Weight < 50 kg = 20 mg enoxaparin/2500 units dalteparin/3500 units tinzaparin daily
Weight 50–90 kg = 40 mg enoxaparin/5000 units dalteparin/4500 units tinzaparin daily
Weight 91–130 kg = 60 mg enoxaparin/7500 units dalteparin/7000 units tinzaparin daily
Weight 131–170 kg = 80 mg enoxaparin/10000 units dalteparin/9000 units tinzaparin daily
Weight > 170 kg = 0.6 mg/kg/day enoxaparin; 75 units/kg/day dalteparin/75 units/kg/day tinzaparin

Figure 10.4 Gross varicose veins are those that are symptomatic, above the knee or associated with phlebitis/oedema/skin changes, immobility for ≥3 days, thrombophilia can be inherited or acquired, long-distance travel is >4 hours. ART, assisted reproductive therapy; BMI, body mass index; LMWH, low-molecular-weight heparin; OHSS, ovarian hyperstimulation syndrome; PPH, postpartum haemorrhage; SLE, systemic lupuserythematosus; SPD, symphysis pubis dysfunction with reduced mobility; VTE, venous thromboembolism. Reproduced with permission from RCOG [1].

Postnatal assessment and management
(to be assessed on delivery suite)

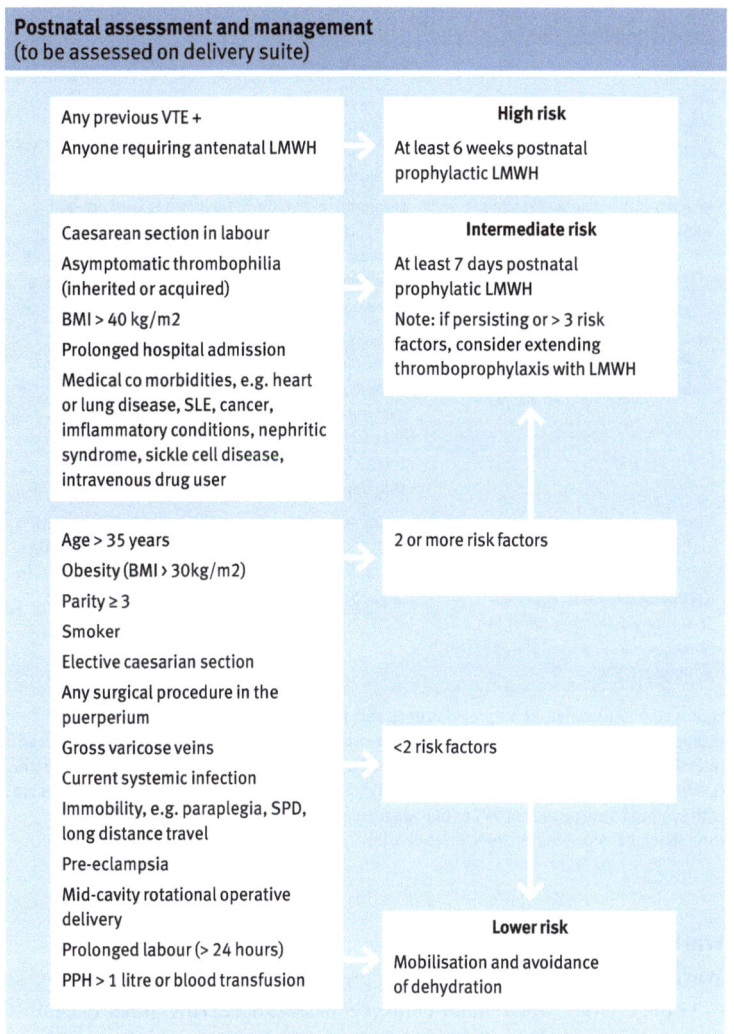

Any previous VTE +

Anyone requiring antenatal LMWH

High risk

At least 6 weeks postnatal prophylactic LMWH

Caesarean section in labour

Asymptomatic thrombophilia (inherited or acquired)

BMI > 40 kg/m2

Prolonged hospital admission

Medical co morbidities, e.g. heart or lung disease, SLE, cancer, imflammatory conditions, nephritic syndrome, sickle cell disease, intravenous drug user

Intermediate risk

At least 7 days postnatal prophylatic LMWH

Note: if persisting or > 3 risk factors, consider extending thromboprophylaxis with LMWH

Age > 35 years

Obesity (BMI > 30kg/m2)

Parity ≥ 3

Smoker

Elective caesarian section

Any surgical procedure in the puerperium

Gross varicose veins

Current systemic infection

Immobility, e.g. paraplegia, SPD, long distance travel

Pre-eclampsia

Mid-cavity rotational operative delivery

Prolonged labour (> 24 hours)

PPH > 1 litre or blood transfusion

2 or more risk factors

<2 risk factors

Lower risk

Mobilisation and avoidance of dehydration

Figure 10.5 Gross varicose veins are those that are symptomatic, above the knee or associated with phlebitis/oedema/skin changes, immobility for ≥3 days, thrombophilia can be inherited or acquired long-distance travel is >4 hours. ART, assisted reproductive therapy; BMI, body mass index; LMWH, low-molecular-weight heparin; OHSS, ovarian hyperstimulation syndrome; PPH, postpartum haemorrhage; SLE, systemic lupus erythematosus; SPD, symphysis pubis dysfunction with reduced mobility; VTE, venous thromboembolism. Reproduced with permission from RCOG [1].

ACCP guidelines for the prevention of VTE in pregnancy

Risk group	Recommendations*
Women with a single episode of VTE associated with a transient risk factor that is no longer present	Clinical surveillance† If the previous event is pregnancy or oestrogen related or there are additional risk factors, antenatal thromboprophylaxis is recommended
Women with a single episode of idiopathic VTE	Antenatal thromboprophylaxis is recommended with LMWH, minidose UFH (5000 IU sc q12h), moderate-dose UFH (UFH sc q12h in doses adjusted to target an anti-Xa level of 0.1–0.3 U/ml) or clinical surveillance† plus postpartum anticoagulants‡
Women with single episodes of VTE and an inherited thrombophilia defect or strong family history of VTE	Antenatal thromboprophylaxis with prophylactic LMWH, intermediate-dose LMWH (e.g. dalteparin 5000 IU sc q12h, or enoxaparin 40 mg sc q12h), minidose UFH (5000 IU sc q12h) or moderate-dose UFH (sc q12h in doses adjusted to target an anti-Xa level of 0.1–0.3 U/ml) plus postpartum anticoagulants‡
For women with antithrombin deficiency or compound heterozygosity for the prothrombin G20210A and Factor V Leiden mutations or homozygosity for these two latter mutations and with a history of VTE	Intermediate-dose LMWH (e.g. dalteparin 5000 IU sc q12h or enoxaparin 40 mg sc q12h) prophylaxis or moderate-dose UFH (sc q12h in doses adjusted to target an anti-Xa level of 0.1–0.3 U/ml)

Figure 10.6 *All women with a previous deep vein thrombosis (DVT) should use graduated elastic compression stockings. † Warfarin for 4–6 weeks with a target international normalised ratio (INR) of 2.0–3.0 with initial unfractionated heparin (UFH) or low-molecular-weight heparins (LMWH) overlap until the INR is ~2.0. ‡ Clinical vigilance and aggressive investigation of women with symptoms suspicious of DVT or pulmonary embolism. SC, subcutaneous; VTE, venous thromboembolism. Adapted from Bates et al [5].

Warfarin

Warfarin is generally avoided during pregnancy and especially during weeks 6–12 of gestation when major embryogenesis is occurring. It has been used in some women during the second trimester (i.e. women with metal heart valves). After delivery, the RCOG suggests that oral anticoagulants may be considered, although only after informing the patient of the need for regular blood monitoring in the first 10 days of treatment [4].

Danaparoid

Danaparoid is a heparinoid (contains heparan sulphate, dermatan sulphate and chondroitin sulphate) that is used mostly in patients with heparin induced thrombocytopenia (HIT) or who develop a skin allergy to heparin. It is given either subcutaneously or intravenously and is monitiored by means of an anti-Xa assay [6].

Fondaparinux

Fondaparinux is a synthetic pentasaccharide which binds to antithrombin. It has only anti-Xa specificity. There is limited use of fondaparinux in pregnancy and evidence suggests that it crosses the placenta.

Nonpharmacological thromboprophylaxis in pregnancy

GECS (British Class II) should be used in all women who receive thrombo-prophylaxis in pregnancy and/or who have a history of a previous VTE. They should continue to wear these for 6–12 weeks after delivery and for up to 2 years in the event of an acute VTE occurring [4].

References

1. Thromboprophylaxis During Pregnancy, Labour and After Vaginal Delivery (guideline no. 37). London: Royal College of Obstetricians and Gynaecologists, 2004. Available at: www.rcog.org.uk/index.asp?PageID=535.

2. Confidential Enquiry into Material and child health (CEMACH) Perinatal mortality 2007: United Kingdon. CEMACH: London, 2009.

3. Royal College of Obstetricians and Gynaecologists. Report of the RCOG Working Party on Prophylaxis Against Thromboembolism in Gynaecology and Obstetrics. London: RCOG, 1995.

4. RCOG. Response to NICE VTE guideline consultation (December 2006). Available at: www.rcog.org.uk/resources/Public/pdf/vte_consultation_response.pdf.

5. Bates SM, Greer IA, Hirsh J, et al. Use of antithrombotic agents during pregnancy: the Seventh ACCP Conference on Antithrombotic and Thrombolytic Therapy. Chest 2004; 126(3, Suppl):627S–644S.

6. Lindhoff-Last E, Kreutzenbeck HJ, Magnani HN. Treatment of 51 pregnancies with danaparoid because of heparin intolerance. Thromb Haemost 2005; 93:63–69.

Index

Note: page numbers in italics refer to figures and text boxes.